Unnecessary Sorrow

A Journalist Investigates
the Life and Death
of His Older Brother
Ordained, Discarded,
Slain by Police

Joe Hight

THE ROADRUNNER PRESS

Help others! End the stigma!

The RoadRunner Press
Oklahoma City, Oklahoma
www.TheRoadRunnerPress.com
Bulk copies or group sales of this book available by
contacting orders@theroadrunnerpress.com

FIRST EDITION, OCTOBER 2019
Printed in the USA

Library of Congress Control Number: 2019936707

Publisher's Cataloging-In-Publication Data
(Prepared by The Donohue Group, Inc.)

Names: Hight, Joe, author.
Title: Unnecessary sorrow : a journalist investigates the life and death of his older brother,
ordained, discarded, slain by police / Joe Hight.
Description: First edition. | Oklahoma City, Oklahoma : The RoadRunner Press, [2019] | Includes
bibliographical references.
Identifiers: ISBN 9781937054991 | ISBN 9781950871025 (ebook)
Subjects: LCSH: Hight, Paul, 1942-2000. | Hight, Joe--Family. | Mentally ill--United States--Biog-
raphy. | Priests--United States--Biography. | Mental illness--Religious aspects--Catholic Church. |
Criminal justice, Administration of--United States. | LCGFT: Biographies.
Classification: LCC RC464.H53 H54 2019 (print) | LCC RC464.H53 (ebk) | DDC 616.890092--dc23

10 9 8 7 6 5 4 3 2 1

*For Father Paul Hight
and all of those courageous people who battle
mental illness daily and whose stories have not been told.
And to Pauline and Wilber Hight,
my Mama and Daddy,
and all families who endure
the painful ordeal of a loved one's illness.*

"I missed my true vocation which was to help people."
—**Paul Hight (1942–2000)**

Prologue

Saintly Beginnings

Some boys dream of comic superheroes—maybe Superman or Batman. Others dream of being star athletes—a Mickey Mantle or a Michael Jordan. Only a few dream of being a saint. Yet there was a time in this country, not so long ago, when that was not so rare a dream, especially if you happened to be born into a Catholic family as my brother and I were.

My own fascination with the saints surfaced in the wake of my First Communion. The year was 1965, and under Sister Elizabeth's watchful eyes, eighteen second-graders and I were lined up for a photograph in the sanctuary of my local church, Saint Mary's Catholic Church in Guthrie, Oklahoma.

We stood in two perfect rows before the ornate altar guarded by two angel sculptures much bigger than we were. Most of the children look solemn for fear of what Sister Elizabeth might do if they smiled: A tug of the hair. An ear pulled. A slap on the back of the head. I had experienced all of those before. Yet there I was on the first row, dressed in my white shirt, dark tie and suit, and black shoes too big for my feet, smiling broadly.

Maybe the smile was for what awaited me when I returned home: a celebratory meal made by my mother, whose made-from-scratch cooking I would fondly remember all my life, and the traditional First Communion present. My gift would be a small illustrated book about the saints. I remember that the book did not look particularly new, probably one of the many hand-me-downs passed on to me, the youngest of seven children. Yet it was new to me, and the stories about the lives that had made these people saints transfixed my young imagination. That First Communion gift changed my dreams. At night, when I stared at the ceiling of the bedroom I shared with my brother Bill, I no longer dreamed of being a superhero or a baseball star, but I did imagine what it would be like to be a true hero, a saint who helped others.

The saints in my little book were mostly from nobility. They were Roman soldiers. They were poor people who performed miracles in life—and even in death. All of them had sacrificed their lives for God and his Church. I admired Saint Joseph, whom I was named after, but I had difficulty imagining that I could ever emulate the father of Jesus. My seven-year-old mind could not grasp the heroic life he had lived. At the time, I had no heroes except for my father and perhaps my oldest brother, Paul, and Saint Joseph was not like my father, an All-State football player and war hero, at least in my eyes. He also was not like Paul, who was only three years from becoming a priest in 1965.

However, one saint did captivate me as a child. The Catholic Church has no shortage of Saint Stephens in its history, with more than thirty now designated as saints. But only one of them is the first Christian martyr, and that is Saint Stephen the Deacon, and his life is the one that spoke to me. His story dates to the first century, the time of Jesus. A nobody appointed by the apostles as one of the first deacons for the Church, he transformed himself into a gifted preacher known for his fiery words in defense of the faith. He eventually drew the attention and ire of the high priests, who hauled him in before them and then ordered that he be stoned to death. Instead of begging for his life, Stephen stood unflinching as the stones were hurled at him. And as the last stone ended his life, he forgave them.

A sixteenth-century Limewood sculpture by German artist Hans Leinberger shows a somber Saint Stephen looking off into the distance as he holds a book, which is said to be a Bible, with three perfectly shaped stones on it. His rosy cheeks and red lips seem untouched by the passage of nearly five hundred years; only his hands appear to have aged through the centuries. I saw the sculpture during a June 2018 visit to the Metropolitan Museum of Art in New York City. Most people had crowded into the museum that day to see "Heavenly Bodies: Fashion and the Catholic Imagination," which was being touted as a "collection to examine fashion's ongoing engagement with the devotional practices and traditions of Catholicism." My only devotion that day, however, was to see this one statue.

As I stood before it, taking in every detail, I couldn't help but feel that Saint Stephen's eyes held a quiet acceptance of his fate—no matter how odd that might sound. For a young Catholic boy in rural Oklahoma in 1965, that's what a true hero looked like. For a man trying to make sense of the life and needless death of his older brother, another Catholic boy reared on the Oklahoma prairie but one who became both a priest and an outcast from his Church because of mental illness, I couldn't help but wonder: Would my oldest brother, Paul, have found acceptance from the Church had he lived in a different time and place?

Books are filled with stories of saints who became martyrs for the Christian faith but whose state of mind we might question today. Their numbers include countless men and women who walked away from civilization to become hermits, most exhibiting what society would now deem strange behavior. I think of Saint Kevin, who settled in the valley of Glendalough in Ireland with the intention of becoming a hermit. When more and more disciples joined him, however, he founded a monastery there instead. One spring day, before his death on June 3, 618, he was found lying on the ground, praying with arms outstretched, similar to how Jesus is depicted on the cross but with a blackbird perched on his hand. That blackbird is said to have laid an egg there, and the man who would become Saint Kevin did not move for weeks until the egg hatched, and the hatchling flew off.

Books are filled with people who acted oddly during their lifetimes but who were deemed worthy of sainthood later and whose contributions to the world are cherished and respected to this day. I say that not because I see my older brother as a candidate for sainthood or to argue that mental illness is a marker for it but to suggest that there have been times in history when odd behavior in a person was not reason enough to cast the person aside, especially in the Catholic Church.

Benedict Joseph Labre, the patron saint of mental illness, was known for his eccentricity in the 1700s. He lived as a beggar in the Colosseum at Rome. The patron saint of priests, John Vianney, spent sixteen to eighteen hours a day in the confessional, but he was also known for his gift of reading minds and souls until his death in 1859. Saint Frances of Rome, patron saint of laity and a known mystic during the 1400s, insisted that she had an angel, visible only to her, as a companion for the last twenty-three years of her life.

Yes, books are filled with people who saw visions or heard voices—but instead of being discarded as my brother was, they became revered, some of them as mystics, some of them as saints. Saint Monica is said to have heard a voice telling her to take her seemingly hopeless son back. Saint Bernadette was taunted by both the Church and authorities because they thought she was hallucinating when she saw visions of Mary telling her to build a chapel in Lourdes, France. The great Joan of Arc heard voices and experienced visions before the nineteen-year-old was burned at the stake May 30, 1431. Today, all three would probably carry the stigma of suffering from schizophrenia or paranoia.

And they are not the only ones whose mental illness also helped shape a saintly life. Saint Francis of Assisi, one of the most beloved of saints, suffered through dark times. Both Saint Dymphna and Saint Catherine of Sienna were thought to have struggled with paranoid schizophrenia or severe mental illness.

And you need to look no closer than Mother Teresa, considered a living saint during her lifetime and known in the Catholic Church as Saint Teresa of Calcutta since her canonization in 2016, to find a woman who lived in a state of deep spiritual pain for almost forty years, a period of time she bemoaned for its sheer loneliness and darkness. Would today's Catholic Church have rejected these men and women, some of history's favorite individuals, some of the Church's greatest saints? Does its own canon law now prevent people who show any sign of mental illness from becoming priests or sisters? Did it or does it seek to reject priests only because they suffer from mental illness, no matter how harmless? Must priests battling depression or other kinds of mental illness live in fear of losing their collar and calling because they have such an illness?

In writing this book about the life and tragic death of my brother, the Reverend Paul Hight, I began to ask such questions. Those and many other questions about the Catholic Church, about our mental health system in the United States, and about the interaction of law enforcement with people struggling with mental illness in this country haunted me throughout the research and writing of this book—so much so that at one point, I wrote on a piece of notebook paper:

We win the battles of our mind and overcome
the challenges of our heart.

The battles and challenges were constant for me in this journey, which lasted more than a decade. During this time, I examined thousands of pages of documents and interviewed family members, Paul's friends, clergy members, police, mental health advocates and officials, and countless others. I also drew upon memories unique to me as Paul's brother. I found that my brother had given away most of his money and possessions during his life, but had kept photographs, articles, report cards, and his own writings, including any writing remotely connected to his life and those he loved and befriended. He left behind countless documents that, in the end, provided clues for the narrative of his life.

For my brother, the battles of the mind were constant. They were hard to win, especially given medication that sometimes impaired him more than the visions that stalked him. His mental illness destroyed his way of living and his dream of being a priest. But others might have contributed to his issues and suffering. Those were people who in the late 1960s and early 1970s upheld the stigma of mental illness—and people who to this day remain stuck in that mind-set in the twenty-first century. Those people still include too many of us and too many of our institutions, with the result being that those who suffer in agony and fear of what the demons will tell them next or, even more frightening, what they will instruct them to do, must live with their fear alone.

I had to battle my own issues after Paul was killed by a police officer in December 2000. I had to battle my own mind telling me I could not do this book; I should not do this book.

As I took on the call to tell Paul's story, I had to battle officials who were slow and sometimes refused to provide records related to my brother as well as some who still refuse to do so. I had to overcome the what-ifs—what if Paul had contributed to his own mental health issues by not taking his medication, what if Paul's clinging to a belief that God and the Catholic Church might someday rescue him from the hell that was his mind also kept him from getting well? I had to overcome anger after my research revealed that Paul might have been expelled as a priest because of his mental illness, and then uncovered that that same mental illness might have been precipitated by a physical illness he suffered in his late teens or early twenties while in the seminary.

This book covers what I believed happened from Paul's birth on December 27, 1942, to his death on December 14, 2000. Although I am a part of the family, I am a minor character to what was transpiring then. The reason: I was born in July 1958, nearly sixteen years after Paul was born. He might have been present at my birth, but I cannot even be sure of that. At the time, Paul had only recently graduated from the two-year Saint Francis De Sales Seminary in Bethany, Oklahoma, and was preparing to leave for San Antonio, Texas, for more high school, college, and the seminary.

Despite this difference in our ages, I cross Paul's path in many and sometimes bizarre ways. Various documents related to Paul's frequent hospitalizations or legal proceedings list my name as a relative along with my father's and mother's. Paul's writings, when he struggled with mental illness, also sometimes listed my name, a discovery that shook me. Early in my life, I wanted to be like Paul, but as a teenager, I came to fear him. His decade of change from 1958 to 1968 turned into decades of uncertainty and tragedy that finally ended in 2000.

In writing a book like this, your mind constantly does battle with you, telling you to stop researching, stop asking questions, stop digging into the past for fear of what you may find or reveal. I have found that in writing about family tragedies and the suffering they cause and the secrets they create, your heart challenges you as well. At times, I cried after writing certain passages of the book. I had nightmares after writing certain others.

I came to realize that we all face challenges of the mind and the heart. My brother Paul most certainly did, and it was his battles that inspired me to write this book. Many other people supported my efforts to write it as well, but my nephew Bryan might have been most instrumental when he wrote in a simple Facebook message: "Uncle Joe, you have to finish the book about Paul."

I told my nephew I would. I couldn't let him down. I couldn't let down Paul or the countless others who suffer with mental illness either. According to the National Institute of Mental Health Disorders, one in four American adults suffers from a diagnosable mental disorder in any given year. That means chances are each and every one of us knows someone—a child, a spouse, a friend, a coworker—who is battling the illness as well as the stigma of mental illness.

We must overcome the stigma. Too many people are misunderstood, misdiagnosed, and mistreated because of their mental illness. Jails are filled with such people. They wander our streets. Some are American heroes returning from wars and conflicts overseas—there is a reason why twenty-two veterans die by suicide each day. And too often, these hurting souls are being ignored by their own family members, who fail to understand why one of their own is acting so strangely or has stepped away from the family. Saint Stephen knew what faced him when authorities dragged him into the pit to be stoned. But right now, millions of people live in a society that throws stones at them, stones shaped by fear and stigma and ignorance. Stones carelessly sculpted into words of news stories that label them or shape narratives that convict them automatically. Stones shaped like bullets that stop the "crazy person" from approaching authorities who are not trained or equipped to handle people with mental illness.

This book is written for those people who have faced what Saint Stephen did in the early days of Christianity but without the knowledge of who or what might cause their ultimate demise.

People like my brother Paul.

Chapter 1

A Family Tragedy

Linda Hight knelt and peered into the water of the stock tank. Catfish swam peacefully below. The small splash that followed changed a family forever.

The day before, Linda and her big brother Paul had visited the water tank, which sat a field away from their family's two-story, white-frame home with no running water in Guthrie, Oklahoma. Dug from the red soil and encased in concrete, the stock tank was separated from the Hight home by a wire fence, just beyond an old oak tree. Wilber Hight had likely gotten the idea for it from one of his many U.S. Soil Conservation Service brochures, a how-to possibly on building a stock tank that could water his cattle and allow him to raise catfish. Once built, however, the tank drew not only cattle but also children as it did on two fateful summer days in 1948.

* * * * *

The Hight family of 1948 was industrious in the can-do way of those who had suffered and survived the Dust Bowl, Great Depression, and

World War II. Wilber and Pauline Hight did what it took to keep their family fed and clothed. They raised catfish in the stock tank, chickens and hogs in the barn, and cattle in a nearby pasture. They had recently attempted a garden, trying to determine what would grow best in Oklahoma's clay soil and unpredictable weather. They had already learned how to store potatoes, freeze corn, and can vegetables, such as beets, to sustain them through the winter.

Theirs was a frugal family. They shopped for clothes in second-hand stores, and Christmas presents were bought at summer sales and stored for months until December 25. And although they had a bank account, Mom never trusted the bank enough to keep all of the family's money there. The Great Depression had taught her that, among other lessons. Instead, she was known to stash a few one-, five-, ten-, and twenty-dollar bills, along with important personal papers, in an old 1800s Wells Fargo safe in the family garage. She also tucked money into various places around the house: dollar bills in books that she thought would never be read, fives under the hardwood floor slats, and Alexander Hamiltons in old hat and shoe boxes in the attic. She never recorded where she placed the money but made a mental note as to where each bill was placed so she could retrieve it should a worthy emergency ever arose. After her death in 1985, it would be years before the house gave up all her hiding places.

Those who knew my mother would say she was even more cautious and protective when it came to her children, although in the end, it was not enough.

The story about what happened on one of those two summer days in 1948 would be told for many years in their small rural community. The stories would vary. When shared, they would often be told in a reverent, hushed tone. A yellowed newspaper story also tried to explain what happened on the second day but not the day before.

That day had ended as all childhood days of summer should end. The highlight of the day found Paul carefully unlatching the gate to the backyard with one hand while clinging with the other to a wooden box. The five-year-old yelled for his baby sister to hurry before their mother called them in for dinner. He was excited, so much so that he might have forgotten his parents' stern warning never to take Linda near the stock tank. It is also possible that it never occurred to him that his sister could be in danger so long as he was with her because, of course, he would protect her from any harm that might arise. He was her older brother. And that was what big brothers did.

Although she was not quite two, Linda was agile and active for her age, with curly auburn hair flecked with gold ringlets that twirled around her forehead and over her ears. She was a fearless little girl, prone to wrestling with the family dog and usually found outside barefoot, playing or riding her tricycle.

The family dog was with them that afternoon as Paul put the wood box in the water and maneuvered it close enough for Linda to crawl into. Their ship was ready to sail. As the catfish swam beneath, Paul pushed Linda about in the makeshift boat. How long the siblings played is lost to history, but at some point, shouts interrupted their play.

"Paul, where are you? Linda . . . Linda!"

It was Mom yelling from the kitchen.

"Where are you two?"

Mom had grown concerned when the house fell quiet, too quiet. Her concern had turned to worry when she looked out the kitchen window and failed to see Paul or Linda in the backyard.

"Mama, we're over here!" Paul yelled.

As he answered, he crawled out of the tank still holding the box. He helped Linda out, and then both children ran for the house, the high grass licking at their heels with the dog barking loudly behind.

Mom frowned as she spotted them.

"Paul, have you been near that tank?"

"Nooo," Paul said.

Paul was not one to lie to his parents, but his father's forceful order not to play with Linda around the stock tank—added to the real possibility of a spanking for disobeying that order—kept the truth untold. Without giving his mother another chance to speak, he declared: "We're hungry! What's for dinner?"

Ignoring his self-serving change of topic, my mother sternly warned again: "You kids better not even think about getting into that tank! Ever!" That was one of two perennial Hight family warnings: Never go near the stock tank, and stay away from the nearby two-lane road. On any other day, Mom also would have told my father immediately what she suspected Paul and Linda had been up to—and have let the children know she planned to do so, but for some reason, Pauline Hight did not do that on this day. Maybe she felt her oldest had gotten the message. Maybe she believed Paul's denial. Maybe she wanted to spare Paul the harsh punishment that surely would have followed otherwise.

Instead, she dropped the subject and issued a different command. "Go get ready for dinner!"

Mom, Paul, and Linda would eat a rare Sunday dinner without our father that evening, because he was off dealing with the birth of a calf. Thus, in the end, no one was there that night to tell about Paul and Linda's escapade.

* * * * *

Our father, Wilber E. Hight, had left his own parents' home in 1933 at the age of sixteen, during the middle of the Great Depression. His father, Irvin, drove him to downtown Guthrie.

"Here's a quarter," his father said. "You'll be back home tomorrow."

"No, I won't."

Wilber never did return to his father's house, preferring to live and work in the Guthrie fire station while he attended high school. At five feet ten inches, he was strapping enough to stop any football player on the opposing line of scrimmage and had admitted more than once that he preferred to knock down forward passes instead of intercepting them. The All-Stater wanted to attend college but lost his football scholarship to Oklahoma A&M in Stillwater, Oklahoma, because of a wrestling injury.

He enlisted in the U.S. Marine Corps, always claiming that he had had a choice in the matter. The way Dad told it, the recruiter claimed so many men wanted to enlist that he could either become a Marine or tear up the enlistment papers and walk away. Never one to walk away from a good fight, my father became a Marine. He rose to the rank of master technical sergeant after being a tough drill sergeant. His deep, bellowing voice could command a room and was ideal for putting the scare into impressionable young men. He loved to tease and was a storyteller too, but he rarely mentioned his time in the Pacific during World War II. The only word I ever heard him use to describe the experience was *Hell*.

He eventually returned to Guthrie, retaining the stern, commanding presence honed in war. He treated my brother Paul as he did the men in his unit. He expected Paul to follow his orders and rebuked him when Paul failed to do exactly as told or expected. If Paul's perceived violation was deemed particularly overt, Dad was not above administering a swat on a five-year-old's bottom. That was rarely necessary because Paul was usually a quietly obedient child. I also suspect my father treated Linda more gently. She had the plump cheeks of a toddler and his daughter's face resembled his wife's. And Mom was the love of my father's life.

They had reconnected in church, her church, while my father was on leave from the *USS Oklahoma*. He had been invited to Mass at Saint Mary's Catholic Church in Guthrie, and he spotted Pauline Kingston when she went up for communion. After Mass, he approached her father, George Albert Kingston, and asked him for her hand in marriage, and then, approval secured, immediately got on one knee to propose to Pauline. She refused at first—she remembered Wilber as being too loud and boastful in high school. However, the confident, uniformed Marine soon won her over. They wed December 21, 1941, in San Diego, California, only a month after Wilber was transferred from the *USS Oklahoma*, which had been sunk December 7 during the Japanese attack on Pearl Harbor in Hawaii. Paul was born a little more than a year later.

My father rose quickly through the ranks, eventually winning the Air Medal before being honorably discharged in 1945. He always said that he left the military so he could focus his life on his wife and family.

His time at war had included brutal battles against the Japanese suicide squads on Guadalcanal in the Pacific Ocean and being rescued in shark-infested waters after his plane went down. According to one family story, he was once positioned behind a machine gun in a bunker on Guadalcanal with fellow Marines when the Japanese launched a series of assaults that kept the Americans firing rounds throughout the night. When dawn broke shortly after the suicide missions ended, my father was the only one alive in the bunker. Years later, when he was safely back home in Oklahoma, thousands of miles from the Pacific battlegrounds of Guadalcanal, that trauma remained with my father, along with the aftereffects of malaria contracted during the war.

A nonpracticing Southern Baptist when he began courting my mother, Dad converted to Catholicism before they wed. And as so often happens with converts, he became a more zealous Catholic than his cradle Catholic wife. In Wilber Hight's house, Sunday was a day of rest no matter what work remained, unless he had a cow calving.

The day of Paul and Linda's trip to the stock tank was a rare cow-calving Sunday, and Dad didn't make it home for dinner. A little after dark, Mom, pregnant with her third child, put the children to bed with a kiss on each forehead and a promise that their father would be home later.

The next morning, when Mom went to wake Paul and Linda, she did so with a reminder. "Daddy will be awake soon, so you better be making your beds because there will be inspections!"

Inspections were as common in the Hight household as they were in the military, and the Hight children, even Baby Linda, knew to take one seriously. Having sounded the warning, my mother noticed that instead of getting out of bed, Paul had already returned to reading his book.

"That includes you, Paul!"

But before Paul could move, a thundering "Good morning! How's the most beautiful woman in the world?" was heard.

Yes, after two children and with a third on the way, my father still felt fortunate to be married to Mom. On this August morning in 1948, his words brought a sunny smile to my mother's face. They also sent Paul and Linda scurrying to put their room in order. Dressed in his

14

usual faded overalls and white T-shirt, Dad pulled on a pair of dirty brown boots with cardboard covering the holes in the soles, finished his breakfast, and headed out to the garden. He had tomatoes to hoe and okra and watermelons to pick before the day became too hot.

"Can you watch Linda this afternoon?" Mom asked on his way out.

Dad nodded, giving her a kiss.

Come lunchtime, Mom called the family in for sandwiches and potatoes and fresh cantaloupe from the garden. Dad ate quickly so he could get back and finish his chores before the sun climbed too high in the sky. The morning hoeing had taken longer than expected, and the unpleasant chore of picking okra remained. On his way out the door, Mom reminded him again that he would need to watch the children while she went grocery shopping that afternoon. Not long after that, Mom left for town.

Temperatures reached nearly 100 degrees Fahrenheit that day. Given the oppressive heat, my father likely told Paul and Linda to go play in the shade under the big oak tree by the family outhouse. And if so his children surely obeyed him.

When my mother returned from the store, the sound of the car pulling in the dirt driveway brought Paul and Linda racing around the house to greet her. Past experience told them that her grocery runs often resulted in a treat for them. This time proved no different.

Dad took a break from picking okra to help carry in the groceries and then returned to the garden. A couple of hours later, the heat having worn him out, he came inside to wash up before settling outside in a lawn chair in the shade for a short break. He had no more gotten comfortable than Mom asked him to watch Paul and Linda so she could start dinner.

A few minutes later, Dad hollered that he needed to check on the livestock. Did he see Mom nod as if to say, *Okay, go?* Did he leave, assuming she was watching the children from the kitchen window? Could he have commanded Paul to watch Linda just to make sure Linda was not unattended before he left? Does it matter anymore? The what-ifs are of no use to anyone now.

Instead, with his father gone and his mother busy with dinner, Paul most likely ran off to do what five-year-olds do when left to their own devices. And with Paul gone, Linda was free to do the same, free to follow her fancy, free to go to the most interesting place on the farm with the family dog. And on this hot August day, that proved to be the stock tank. Maybe Linda had wanted to see those catfish with the big whiskers again; maybe she wanted to feel the cool water on her fingertips.

The loud barking was what caused my mother to eventually look out the window. Where was Wilber? Where was Paul? Where was Linda? Were the children out in the pasture with their father? Why did that dog keep barking?

Unable to see anyone, she stepped to the screen door and yelled: "Wilber, do you know where the kids are?"

Paul heard her immediately. "I'm here! I'm here!"

Dad had also heard her call and started for the house.

They reunited in the backyard by the old oak tree—each looking at the other with puzzled expressions, each asking the same question: "Where's Linda?"

Paul shrugged his shoulders when asked.

The barking continued.

Yelling their daughter's name over and over as loud as they could, Mom and Dad took off in opposite directions looking for her. Paul trailed his mother as she ran frantically to the garden. Dad rushed to the pasture just beyond the old oak tree. In the distance, he could hear the faint sound of his wife calling for Linda.

As he approached the stock tank, he noticed a wood box nearby and wondered why it was there. He drew closer and spotted something pink floating in the water. Dread filled his heart. He broke into a run, and in the seconds that must have felt like hours, he reached the tank only to find Baby Linda face down in the water.

The tortured cry that followed could be heard all the way across the pasture to the garden: "Noooooooooo!"

Mom and Paul found him cradling Linda's limp little body in his arms. He had been too late. The precocious little girl with the infectious laugh and curious nature was gone, dead before her second birthday. Dad carried Linda's body to the house. He had seen many lifeless bodies during World War II. He had lost many buddies there too. But nothing had prepared him for this.

Children are not supposed to die before their parents. It is such a rare and unnatural occurrence, there is not even a word for a parent who has lost a child as there is for a widow or widower. The emotional pain must have been excruciating, but my father stayed calm, as the Marines had trained him to do in times of crisis, for the sake of his pregnant wife and son.

Dad knew what he had to do, and he surrendered to all the little tasks that come with a death in the family. He called the funeral home and told them Linda had drowned in the stock tank. The funeral home director called the sheriff as he was required to do, and then both men headed for the Hight place. The sheriff quickly realized Linda's death was a tragic accident. He had seen it happen before: One parent thinks the other is watching the child, and the child wanders off. The stories didn't always end with such finality, but too often they did.

The following Wednesday at ten o'clock in the morning, as the rest of the country was mourning the death of New York Yankees great Babe Ruth, the Mass of Angels was held for Linda Ann Hight at the family church, followed by her burial in the local cemetery. That night found Paul in the room he had shared with his sister staring at the ceiling, bewildered by all that had happened. Across the room, Linda's bed was neatly made but empty.

In the living room, Dad rocked back and forth in his rocker as he struggled to understand why such a tragedy had befallen his family. Why had his little girl been snatched away? Why was God punishing his family when he had already suffered so much during the war? Searching for someone to blame and finding no one, he turned the guilt inward, on himself, on his wife, and on his only remaining child.

Mom had told him about her suspicions that Paul had taken Linda to the water tank the day before the accident. She confessed to being upset with herself for not having pressed the matter, for not having found out the truth. If she had made more of a fuss, she whispered, would Linda have still returned to the tank on her own?

They would never know.

Sitting in the dark, thinking about what might have been, Wilber opened the Bible in a last-ditch hope that something in it could somehow explain why this loss had happened to his family, the ones he was supposed to protect. He would look for signs. He had taught his family to do the same. Whether he found one that night, we don't know, but eventually he put the Bible down and walked upstairs to Paul's room, looking for answers or maybe someone to blame.

"How could you have taken your sister to the water tank when you had been told not to over and over again?"

No explanation Paul could give would ever be enough for my father.

The tragedy that had befallen the Hight family would cause lingering sorrow and guilt for the three who remained for the rest of their lives. They held their feelings deep inside, rarely mentioning that day unless specifically asked. My father would forgive his oldest son for what had happened that day, but he could never forget. Dad and Paul would live with the loss of Baby Linda, often seemingly in conflict with each other.

And in the wake of the loss of his daughter, my father changed. He looked for a way to atone for the drowning. He searched the Bible many more times in the future for answers. Did any of the words in the Good Book bring solace or ease his mind? Did any of the verses or Bible stories reveal how a family made it through the pain of such a loss?

Dad became a more devout Catholic, building a beautiful wooden altar in memory of his oldest daughter for his parish church. His penance, Paul's penance, would heal and restore the Hight family. Because from that brief exchange between father and son on the night of Linda's burial, Paul's answer to righting this horrible wrong became clear: He would become the perfect priest.

Chapter 2

First Signs

The cherrywood china cabinet was the centerpiece of the Hight dining room in the family's new red brick home east of Guthrie. Mom had positioned the piece of furniture to keep the 1960s air conditioner, which kept part of the house cool during hot summers, from dripping water onto the porch outside and on occasion inside onto her dining room floor.

Mom and Dad had moved to the one-story home in the early 1960s, and the move meant they no longer lived in sight of where their baby girl had drowned more than a decade before. Dad, with help from family and others, then built the house on three acres of land that adjoined the home of Mom's parents. Mom said we made the move so she could watch her folks as they grew older.

By the time we moved in, we were a typical Catholic family of the times with four sons—Paul, John, Bill, and me—and two daughters, Susan and Marilyn. The family had become large enough that Dad was known to recite our names in order of birth to get the child he wanted. "*PaulSusanJohnBillMarilynJoe*, you come here right now!" The refrain was heard loud and often, because our father also used it to summon his children in one fell swoop or to ensure that all of us were listening to him when he had something to say. Missing, always loudly missing, however, was Linda, who would have been a teenager by then.

Mom, Dad, and Paul carried her with them always—and somehow the rest of us, who had come after Linda, sensed that. My mother kept the story of her first daughter's death in an old cigar box, tucked inside a drawer in the cherry china cabinet, not that they needed it to remember.

The yellowed clipping had been hastily cut from the *Guthrie Daily Leader*. The newspaper carried a short article about Olen Williams resigning as head football coach of Central High School in Oklahoma City, Oklahoma, to become a sporting goods salesman. And below that, an ad, with a photo of a homely Pennsylvania woman with a square jaw, promoting a new brand of bran cereal from Kellogg's. The flip side of the page included a weather forecast calling for highs reaching possibly 100 degrees Fahrenheit that day.

Under the weather, the front-page headline read, "Child's Play Ends in Death." Six paragraphs told the story of how Linda's little adventure had ended in tragedy. It read in part:

> While both of the young parents were busy with evening chores, Linda Ann fell into a tank used for watering stock and was drowned.
>
> The mother noticed the infant was absent from where she had been playing in the yard, but thought she probably had accompanied her father, who had gone after livestock in a nearby pasture.
>
> When he returned, and it was discovered the infant hadn't accompanied him, a search was launched, resulting in the finding of her body in the tank by Hight.

Linda died August 16, 1948, and was buried in a family plot my parents bought for $160, the same plot where they would someday be buried, along with my brother Paul. The newspaper clipping, like the memories, followed us to the new house, but other than that, Linda's death was rarely mentioned in the Hight household, although my mother was once heard to say that Linda was in Heaven.

Linda's death left her older brother, as well as the brothers and sisters who followed after her death, wondering who she might have been had she lived. Would she have followed their father's example and become the athlete of the family? Would she have been the one to care for her younger brothers and sisters when their mother couldn't, instead of the next oldest daughter, Susan? Would Marilyn have been the youngest child instead of me?

Had Linda lived, the Hight family would have had three boys and three girls, and a seventh might have been one too many, even for a good Catholic family. Years later, Mom would say she and Dad agreed to have one more child after watching John's First Communion. Had Linda lived, would that decision have been different? Five of us children had never known Linda, yet we knew our lives had been touched by her absence in ways we could and could not imagine.

And then there was Paul. At the age of ten, he made our mother a card out of notebook paper that read:

> *Dear Mother,*
> *I love you very much and I will ask Jesus and Mary to*
> *love you alway(s).*
> *Paul Wilber Hight*

On the neatly folded note he put a sticker of Mary and Joseph leading a young Jesus through the street. Jesus's right arm is stretched outward. Did Paul see himself being led in the same direction with his own mother and father behind him?

His parents and Grandma Kingston, a devout Catholic with Irish roots, certainly encouraged Paul to consider the priesthood. By age fourteen, Paul was living at Saint Francis de Sales Seminary in Bethany, Oklahoma, a suburb just west of Oklahoma City, Oklahoma, the state capital. At that time in 1958, the dioceses of Oklahoma City, Dallas, Amarillo, Austin, Galveston, Corpus Christi, and El Paso were all in the Archdiocese of San Antonio, Texas, headed by Archbishop Robert E. Lucey. A Los Angeles native, Lucey was best known for having integrated the Catholic schools in his archdiocese in 1953, a year before the U.S. Supreme Court's *Brown v. Board of Education* ruling that ended legal segregation in public schools.

A two-year school for freshmen and sophomores, Saint Francis de Sales Seminary was a junior, or minor, seminary where teenage boys could continue their studies and begin a path toward the priesthood. The place was run by priests from the Congregation of the Mission, or Vincentian Fathers or Lazarists, a community of Roman Catholic priests and brothers founded by Saint Vincent de Paul in 1625 and known for evangelization of the poor and formation of future clergy as well as being strict rule makers.

In those days, Paul was a bookish, sensitive, and reserved young man, much like his mother in disposition. But one old friend recalled that Paul was also "very influenced by what his father had to say—and wanted to make him happy." Paul was one of a class of twenty to thirty teenage boys from Oklahoma and parts of Texas, most of whom were probably there at the behest of their parish priest. In one school photo, Paul stands at attention in the front row as if he were in the military where his father had so thrived. Black shoes cover the size thirteen feet that would eventually support his height. Through dark-rimmed, round glasses, he smirks shyly at the camera.

After completing two years at the minor seminary, at the age of only sixteen—an age when most young men are still living at home and thinking about driving, dating, and drinking, the same age that his father left home a generation before—Paul boarded a Greyhound bus for the almost five-hundred-mile trip to San Antonio to continue his high school studies. Dad never returned to live at home again after his exodus. Paul would not either.

In San Antonio, Paul attended Saint John's Seminary, a high school also run by the Vincentians. Established in 1915 by Bishop John Shaw, the thirteen-acre site south of downtown San Antonio included a high school and a college, a rarity in the United States. Thirty-one students and Paul comprised his class on a campus of one hundred students. Paul lived in a three-story dormitory attached to a classroom building. He followed a regimented life of study, sports, and worship, not unlike the life he would have lived at home had he stayed.

His day began with a 6:00 a.m. wake-up call, followed by chapel at the adjacent Mission Nuestra Senora de la Purisima Concepcion de Acuna. Mission Concepcion, as Paul and his classmates knew it, was built in 1755, the oldest unrestored stone church in the country. A painting of Jesus ascending to heaven overlooks the chapel's simple altar. And, at the time, the minor-league San Antonio Missions baseball team played in the stadium across the street.

Breakfast was followed by chapel, followed by classes in history, Latin, and other typical high school subjects. Most afternoons were reserved for study; dinner was served promptly at six o'clock. The students ate separately from the priests, who were served by students at a long communal table. Evenings were for student activities, with lights out at 10:00 p.m. sharp. The boys slept in a long, barrackslike room with a bathroom at the end. The students' only time off came on Wednesdays and Sundays when they were allowed to take a public bus or school van to a nearby bowling alley or downtown. The boys abided by rules that included no smoking or chewing of gum, maintaining good hygiene, keeping their grades up, and always showing up prepared and on time.

The rules included no studying—even under the covers—after 10:00 p.m. Students were known to drink large amounts of water the night before a test so they had an excuse to go to the lighted bathroom, where they would continue their studying. But they did so at their own peril. Breaking a rule was punishable by expulsion. One of Paul's classmates was kicked out of school just weeks before graduation for chewing gum. Other graduates from his class went on to become priests, lawyers, social workers, and doctors—as for the fellow expelled for chewing gum, well, he became a dermatologist in Florida.

May 1960 was Paul's time to graduate from Saint John's, but he never made it to graduation. *The Eaglet*, published on graduation day at Saint John's Seminary, featured both the photographs of the 1960 class as well as member biographies written by their classmates. The black-and-white photos were mostly profiles of graduates, all wearing white shirts, dark ties, and coats. Some smiled. Some did not. In his photo, Paul can be seen shyly smirking again at the camera. He wears his usual dark-rimmed glasses, and his hair is combed to one side with a noticeable cowlick in the back, a trait that plagues many of the Hight men.

The booklet is dedicated to three graduates who would not be attending graduation exercises on May 26, 1960, including one whose father had died unexpectedly. The other two were described as the booklet's "own editor, Mr. Richard Kramer, and Mr. Paul Hight, both of whom illness will prevent them [sic] from attending."

No details about either student's illness was given, and back home, no mention was ever made of why Paul missed his own graduation that I recall. Could it have been the first sign that Paul was beginning a lifelong struggle with mental illness? Or was he down with the flu or another common, maybe contagious, ailment that made attending graduation impossible?

Whatever my brother's health problem, the illness was not deemed important enough to include in his biography in the *Eaglet*. Indeed, Paul's biography is one of the shortest, only five paragraphs long, the same length as one written about a student who had attended the seminary for only a year. As with the others, the headline carried his name in all capital letters, identified him as being from the Diocese of Oklahoma City–Tulsa, and noted that he had performed in "numerous plays and operettas" at Saint Mary's School in Guthrie and sang a solo for the bishop at his confirmation. It went on to read:

> After grade school Paul entered Saint Francis Seminary in Bethany, Oklahoma, for his freshman and sophomore years. As a junior, Paul came to Saint John's.
>
> During his two years here, he has held various jobs, as bell ringer and light checker. Paul likes all sports but especially basketball. His hobbies are hunting and fishing, playing dominoes, and a new one, penny collecting.

When he is home, Paul works on the farm.

His favorite foods are pork chops and pumpkin pie.

There is one unusual event in Paul's life that is particularly interesting. In the summer before his junior year, Paul entered a fishing contest. Well, Paul caught the biggest fish. It was a channel catfish weighing nine-and-a-half pounds. He also won the prize and that prize, of all things, was a case of beer.

Paul had indeed caught a record catfish of almost ten pounds while home the summer after his junior year, to the amazement of us all. The catch prompted Dad to make an unexpected stop at the Rock Way Bar on our way home.

"Paul, get out with your fish and come with me," Dad said after pulling into the gravel parking lot in front of the bar. "The rest of you stay in the car."

Paul dutifully grabbed the catfish and marched in lockstep with Dad into the darkly lit tavern. We didn't find Dad entering a bar particularly shocking. He had friends in all kinds of places. When his youngest brother, Lawrence, came to town, they were known to frequent a dive or two, local holes with patrons that Dad was known to describe as being "rougher than a cob," a term for tough, abrasive men that comes from the days when people used corncobs instead of toilet paper in outhouses during the Great Depression. Dad and especially Mom never admitted to having used corncobs in such a manner, but my father was known to use the term when describing a certain caliber of people. What he was not known to do was bring his underage children into a bar. Once inside, he loudly announced to the bar patrons in attendance, "Look at what my son caught!"

There are few things more appreciated in an Oklahoma bar, then or now, than a big catfish. The bar patrons erupted in resounding cheers, and then everybody crowded around to see and admire Paul's catch. My shy brother probably was proud to have caught a fish that impressed not only our father but also our father's friends, but photographs snapped of Paul and his big fish that day show a teenage boy struggling to smile while holding the catfish.

As for winning a prize? Or setting a record? *The Eaglet* biography must have been embellished. Paul did catch a large fish that summer, the photograph and family lore attest to that, but neither makes mention of any contest or, for that matter, his winning a case of beer.

As noted in his *Eaglet* biography, the tallest Hight son tried playing basketball in high school but was too clumsy to continue. The image of a jock never fit Paul anyway. He possessed the gentleness of his mother, who every night before going to sleep could be found kneeling bedside in quiet prayer. My mother never told anyone what she was praying about, but Linda, who with her chubby cheeks resembled one of those cherubs in heaven, surely must have been in her thoughts.

The Eaglet biography makes no mention either of Paul's poem the "Herald of God" being published in the National High School Poetry Association's Anthology of High School Poetry or that he liked to write and tell stories. The award-winning poem was lost to the pages of time, but the poem's existence reveals that my older brother had a gift for writing and storytelling. It was a talent he shared with his father.

However, except for a deep, bellowing voice and occasional ornery behavior, it might have been one of the only qualities that Paul and Dad both possessed.

Chapter 3

The Men Behind the Collar

Familiarity breeds contempt, they say. At the very least, it can dispel any delusions about a person. Paul was studying to become a priest at a time when the clergy were still universally held in high regard in this country—and not just by Catholics. It was a time of routines that American Catholics shared from coast to coast: They ate fish on Fridays. They attended Mass on Sunday morning. Women wore hats in church, and men did not. And Mass was celebrated in Latin.

Comfort comes from such routine. Children are said to both crave and thrive on it. The Hight family followed those routines.

They dressed in their finest clothes and filed into the same pew with the tarnished brass plate No. 73 for ten o'clock Mass at Saint Mary's, a parish founded after the 1889 Land Run that brought settlers from all over the world to Oklahoma. The church was intended to become the territory's first cathedral until Oklahoma City and not Guthrie became the state capital.

In the Hight pew, Dad usually sat on the end, whittling away at the dirt underneath his fingernails with his pocketknife or using it occasionally to pick at his teeth when Mom wasn't looking. Our mother sat beside him, followed by the children, one by one, from oldest to youngest.

After Mass, parishioners would often gather outside to discuss the news and visit. The Hights were among those who stayed afterward. Often, they could be overheard talking to the priest or friends about the latest news from Paul and how many years remained until he would become a priest, one of the few to ever come out of this small parish.

Their Sunday church obligation fulfilled, the Hights would head home, where Dad's next task was to command the Hight children to sit on the couch for his weekly lecture. Paul probably had to endure many of those alone after Linda's passing.

My father used the time to impart "words of wisdom" with the fist-clenching and pacing of the Baptist preachers he had grown up listening to as a child. He imagined himself another Knute Rockne, only Dad was intent on inspiring his children instead of the University of Notre Dame football team. (My father knew all about Notre Dame and Knute Rockne because back then most Catholics—and most of America—watched the games on their black-and-white televisions. The Irish still draw ire in Oklahoma for ending the forty-seven-game winning streak of the Sooners with a 7-0 upset victory in 1957 in Norman.)

His lectures were heavy on clichés and the positive-thinking platitudes of Norman Vincent Peale. "You were *born* to be a leader!" he would bellow. "You should always be ready to *lead* others!" He never failed to remind us that would not be easy: "You have to *pay* the fiddler if you want to dance—it takes hard work to achieve one's goals and overcome obstacles."

Dad was a self-described "bull-shooter" from a long line of bull-shooters, who were known to use stories to make their points in their frequent but friendly arguments. The former Marine, however, limited his use of the more common profanities for when he was angry or around other bull-shooters, softening his vocabulary around his children but especially when his wife, who rarely cursed, was within earshot. That said, my father was a bull-shooter who did not fear repetition or pray at the altar of variety. Instead, each Sunday morning, he repeated the same stories, truisms, and refrains until they became filed in the minds of his children as deeply as their childhood prayers.

The Hights' weekly Sunday routine continued with a big lunch of fried chicken, meatloaf, or roast beef, served with fresh corn, tomatoes, fried okra or other vegetables, watermelon, cantaloupe, and a dessert, usually bread pudding, rice pudding, or a frosted pan cake. My mother was a good cook who became an expert at serving large family meals, which she finished in the quiet of the kitchen during Dad's lectures. The appetizing aromas coming from the kitchen might have occasionally brought those talks to a quicker conclusion, but not often. Dad took this weekly wisdom-sharing time seriously, and the one topic that he returned to again and again had to do with making the right decision about what to do with your one and only life.

Paul was destined to become a priest, but Dad's other sons had yet to choose. They had a choice: Enlist in the military after high school or go to college. "You should enlist in the Navy or the Army, but not the Marine Corps because it'll be too tough for you," Dad always said. "I would suggest enlisting in the service [over college] because you need discipline in your life."

The family bull-shooter was not above using reverse psychology. He cajoled his children to enlist so they would do the exact opposite. He mastered the art so well that one could be forgiven for wondering if he was bull-shooting or being candid when it came to the question of what we should do with our lives. Either way, his system worked: All three sons chose college over the military. As for Paul, well, he was studying to become a priest, a position of untold pride for his parents, his siblings, and the rest of the extended family.

Before the sexual abuse scandal rocked the Roman Catholic Church in the 1990s, the priesthood was considered the pinnacle of success for the oldest son of any Catholic family. Few honors were greater than having your local priest to dinner or as a regular visitor in your home. The Hight children were accustomed to finding a priest asleep on the couch in the living room or sitting across the table from them at dinner. The priests from Saint Mary's—from one who became bishop of Kansas City, Missouri, to an old Irish priest to a political activist who later became a park ranger to a fun-loving pastor—were counted among the

Hight family's best friends. As a result, Paul regularly saw and came to know the men behind the collar before he ever donned one himself.

After early retirement from the Air Logistics Center, Dad began to teach at the local job corps for disadvantaged youth. He still tended his garden, but he also began to build furniture. He turned the red barn behind the east Guthrie house into a carpentry shop where he would disappear for hours. He became quite a proficient carpenter; he was soon joined by Father E. Joseph Thompson, a priest who had a knack for making people angry with his sermons. (During one sermon in which Father Thompson denounced the U.S. president, a parishioner reportedly stomped out of the church, slamming the doors behind him, never to return.)

Father Thompson and my father built items for that very same church, from a chair for the priest to a large wooden altar. Dad went on to work with dark walnut, making furniture so heavy that two to three strong people were required to carry the pieces, which included bookcases, a desk, a chest with a hutch, and a chest of drawers.

Later in life, Dad gave pieces of his handmade furniture to his children—all his children expect Paul.

My father's reasoning: "Paul wouldn't take care of it anyway or he would just give it away to some bum who happened to ask. I can't bear to think of that happening to something I built with my own hands."

Chapter 4

The Tumultuous Sixties

After Paul graduated from Saint John's High School in 1960, he traveled again by Greyhound bus to Saint Louis, Missouri, more than nine hundred miles north of San Antonio. Still a teenager, still far from home, still influenced by the Vincentian Community, he followed his calling—not knowing that a movement was about to transform the Catholic Church and everyone associated with it.

Before, in January 1959, Pope John XXIII had called for the Second Vatican Council as a means of spiritual renewal for the Catholic Church. A pope had not called for such a council in nearly a hundred years. After much planning, an estimated two thousand to twenty-five hundred bishops—and thousands of observers, nuns, auditors, and laypeople—attended four council sessions at Saint Peter's Basilica in Rome between 1962 and 1965. Vatican II, as it was also called, and the sixteen documents it produced rocked the world.

For some Catholics who had been taught that the pope was infallible, such a council wasn't deemed needed any more than input from the laity was desired. But Vatican II aimed to change all that as it called for the Catholic Church to open itself more to the world and the changing times, including recognizing and communicating with other religions. In English-speaking countries, the Church began to use English instead of Latin for the Mass. The liturgy, the way the Mass was celebrated, was updated. And most important, the Church gave new roles to laypeople. As Pope John XXIII told the council:

> The Church should never depart from the sacred treasure of truth inherited from the Father. But at the same time, she must ever look to the present, to the new conditions, and the new forms of life introduced in the modern world.

Some Catholics welcomed the changes. Others railed against them. In the end, Vatican II created a deep-rooted schism in the Church that continues to this day between more conservative clergy and Catholics and progressive Catholics more willing to embrace change in the Church. The changes also had an impact on the men studying to be priests in the 1960s, especially on young seminarians such as Paul.

Paul entered Cardinal Glennon College in Saint Louis one year after the pope's declaration and two years before the meetings began in Rome. The college was then part of Kenrick Seminary, also known as Saint Louis Preparatory Seminary. Its roots date to 1818, when the Vincentians founded the first seminary west of the Mississippi River in Perryville, Missouri. The seminary remained there until 1842, when Bishop Peter Richard Kenrick moved it to Saint Louis. Five years later, Kenrick became an archbishop.

The seminary officially became Kenrick Seminary with the move to the site of a former convent in the late 1800s. Moved again by a future cardinal, Archbishop John J. Glennon, the seminary eventually became a combination high school and college.

By the time Paul moved to San Antonio, Joseph E. Ritter, another archbishop who became a cardinal, had established a four-year high school for clerical and nonclerical students, a four-year college, and a theologate, a seminary that teaches theology to future priests. All were vital for any young man wanting to become a priest, and the college was already transforming itself because of Vatican II. In an editorial in October 1962, the college's student newspaper/magazine, *The Cassock*, opined:

> One of the most eagerly awaited results of the present Ecumenical Council is the increased importance and participation [of] the laity in ecclesiastical affairs. Most churchmen will admit that in the past the value of interested laymen in the Church has been greatly underestimated, but few have either been in a position or seen fit to do anything about it.

The editorial announced that an advisory board had been appointed at the seminary. It was comprised of all men, including officials of the college, priests, and monsignors who held key roles in the archdiocese, pastors, an attorney, a doctor, and "Mr. Leo J. Wieck, a gentleman active in archdiocesan affairs before and since his retirement." The board was tasked with advising students, creating policies, and working with the community to advance the college and improve relations.

At Cardinal Glennon College, Paul took general classes in religion, philosophy, English, Greek, Latin, education, music, and theology, making mostly As and Bs. He also took more specific classes, such as "Parochial Law," "Art of Confessional Practice," "Ministry and Liturgical Celebration," and other Church law classes.

He was a good test-taker and earned a certificate of eminent merit/ maxima cum laude for distinguished proficiency in Latin from the Association for Promotion of Study of Latin, scoring a 110 out of a possible 120 on a nationwide Latin examination. The only stain on his academic performance was in the canon law classes, in one of which he made a C+.

When not studying or attending class, Paul sang in the choir, acted in plays—one time as an old man with a cane—and worked on *The Cassock*, becoming a contributing writer. In that same 1962 edition, he wrote in a satirical essay called "Backfire" about the end of the semester and a return trip home. He pointed to the continuing tension and influence exerted by his father.

> Cram, cram history, speech, Greek, English exams. Cram, cram suitcases.
>
> At the bus station, there would be bums all over, smoke-filled bus, over-perfumed lady with overworking mouth, jabbering, jabbering about some girl who knew this boy who had a girl, and what a hussy—smashed by a big bulk of rotundity against the side of the bus.
>
> Oh, my aching back. Now going home—ah . . . rest.
>
> However, after arriving home late, to be awakened early the next morning.
>
> "Paul . . . What do you say we go out and see Daddy?"
>
> "Daddy—work? But Mom, I'm pooped."
>
> "But Paul, that's all he's talked about—about how glad he'd be to see good ole Paul. Now you're going to disappoint him."
>
> "No, I guess not, but you know good and well why he's looking forward to seeing 'good ole Paul!' "
>
> "Now, Paul. He just likes you."
>
> "I know, I know."
>
> [I] was trapped, without any labor unions to demand better working conditions—trapped in the narrow confines of our family car, which, greatly to my discomfort, had never swerved from its path to some bare plot of ground, my Dad, and w-o-r-k.

But Mom's cajoling soon had Paul changing out of his dress clothes into work ones that she had brought along, just in case. Paul wrote that Dad had also added a little bull-shooting request as an added incentive.

It was bull-shooting that Paul might have embellished on in his satirical essay:

"My dear son, by reason of your eminent experience in the seminary, you have been chosen for a most distinguished and holy project, and I, in the name of the entire Hight family, wish to give you the first impetus, that initial helping hand . . . with this shovel. Here."

The whole experience caused Paul to write:

The seminary's not so bad after all.

* * * * *

Paul's eight years in Saint Louis would see tumultuous changes, not only in the American Catholic Church but also in the country. The decade included the assassinations of Robert F. Kennedy and Martin Luther King Jr., the Vietnam War, the civil rights movement, war protests, and the hippie counterculture movement. One Oklahoma priest described 1968 as the "wildest year of the century." But it was what happened on June 5, 1968, that proved particularly agonizing for Dad.

"We need to go to church to pray now," Dad announced, choking up. "Robert Kennedy was shot this morning. Martin Luther King was killed just a couple of months ago. This world is going to hell, and we have to do something about it!"

His way to do that was to pray.

As the family left for Saint Mary's Church, black-and-white images of the chaos that had ensued after the assassination of Kennedy at the Ambassador Hotel that morning in Los Angeles flashed across the TV screen. Dad would later snap photos of that same screen in happier times during live TV coverage of Neil Armstrong and Buzz Aldrin landing on the moon for the first moonwalk in July 1969. But on that June evening in 1968, he was focused only on getting his family to church. He led his children into Saint Mary's, away from the family's usual pew and toward the front of the church. Candles flickered on the altar. Other men, women, and children were already there, scattered in pews throughout the darkened church—some praying, some sitting in shock, some crying silently. My parents, deeply troubled by the events of the day, knelt to pray. They did not notice or comment as their children filed in beside them in no particular order. All normality, all the routines that had held their life together for so long, were abandoned that night. When they left the church that night, they did so in silence.

Neither my father nor my mother ever talked about that evening again. Somehow it was as if in the face of our country's unspeakable loss, God had lifted the trouble from their souls.

The troubles of the time were not unique to the big cities of Detroit or Los Angeles or Chicago. Paul's small hometown of Guthrie, which in 2019 still numbers only a little more than ten thousand souls, was also going through troubled times. Over the years, the town had self-segregated into two parts: white Guthrie and what was called colored town. Schools were segregated. Another section of Guthrie became known as Little Africa for its high proportion of blacks. Even the town's two parks were divided according to color: Highland Park for whites and Mineral Wells Park for blacks. It would be 1967 before the last all-black school, Faver High School, was closed as part of the town's integration efforts.

Away in Saint Louis at school, Paul was mostly insulated from the troubles at home. He continued his studies and work at *The Cassock*, where he eventually became managing editor. One lead editorial run under his watch called "Crucifixion in Cell Eight" recounts an evening spent in the Saint Louis Police Department's cell No. 8. That cell provided the homeless a night out of the cold and the next morning a "king's breakfast of bread, a generous hunk of bologna, and hot coffee to prepare them for their nearing departure. The cell is home for a night, but the chilling world awaits them at daybreak."

The editorial describes a drawing of Jesus dying on the cross that had been drawn three decades earlier on the back wall of the cell. No one knew how or why it was drawn, just that the art was a "feat of difficult sketching" and had been there since the 1930s. An elderly janitor at the jail told of "a man kneeling, in the posture of prayer, in front of the wall. When he returned shortly, the man was gone and Christ was on the wall." Known as the "Holy Cell," the cell with the drawing went unused for years, but police continued to keep a light on it at night. Eventually, the drawing was cut from the cell wall and placed on display in the police library. By 1970, half a million people were reported to have viewed the cell mural.

During his time at Cardinal Glennon College, Paul grew out of his awkward teens into a handsome young man, with short sandy-blond hair cropped around his ears and dark-rimmed glasses he wore for his nearsightedness. His face still resembled that of his mother, yet he now had his father's strong jaw. At nearly six feet, four inches tall, he was easily the tallest Hight family member, with a lanky body that went with his big feet.

For the first time in his life, he exuded confidence. He smiled broadly in photographs. He laughed openly in public and began to tell stories as his bull-shooter father had done for so many years. And he made friends. One fellow seminarian at the time, Jack Petuskey, who became one of the most respected pastors in Oklahoma as Father John Petuskey, gave Paul a photo on which he wrote:

> *Dear Paul,*
> *Your joy and apostolic love have been an example to me. I look forward to being with you in Oklahoma where we can work together!*

In 1964, Paul earned a bachelor's degree from Cardinal Glennon College. Four years later, he received a bachelor of divinity degree from Saint Louis University; he attended Kenrick Seminary in Saint Louis while going to summer school at Fordham University in New York and the University of Oklahoma in Norman.

At the time, Paul seemed destined for Europe for more education, possibly even Rome, where future bishops are trained. Oklahoma City–Tulsa Bishop Victor J. Reed took great pride in his priests and in furthering their education. Paul, having embraced the spirit of Vatican II and believing its changes would have a positive impact on the Church, would have been an ideal candidate. My brother was eager to spread the word of God with this new wind at his back.

In April 1966, the words of Pope Paul VI, who succeeded Pope John XXIII after his death in June 1963, must have resonated with Paul:

> Whatever were our opinions about the Church's various doctrines before its conclusions were promulgated, today our adherence to the decisions of the Council must be whole hearted and without reserve; it must be willing and prepared to give them the service of our thought, action, and conduct. The Council was something new; not all were prepared to understand and accept it. But now the conciliar doctrine must be seen as belonging to the magisterium of the Church and, indeed, be attributed to the breath of the Holy Spirit.

The future must have seemed so full of promise for the Oklahoma boy so far from home and from the tragedy of that hot August afternoon some twenty years earlier.

Traveling home to Oklahoma, Paul looked into a sky washed clean by a thunderstorm that had pelted the area with hailstones and heavy rain. A tornado watch had been issued, but none had materialized. Instead, a brilliant rainbow had formed and stretched across the horizon.

"You see that," Paul said, pointing at the rainbow. "That rainbow is God's promise to us. We will never again see the forty days of flooding that destroyed the earth. God cleansed the earth of its sins that time but made a promise to all of us that He will always be with us, and He will always protect us. We must believe in Him always. We must always evangelize that there will be a rainbow after a storm. God always gives us hope."

Paul had completed twelve years of training that would culminate in not only a grand ordination to celebrate the beginning of his priesthood but also the beginning of a storm that would descend and consume his life.

Chapter 5

The Number Eight

The number eight might seem to have no particular significance. It follows the lucky seven. No one places any special significance on an eighth anniversary. It is not divisible by five. But years ending in eight have repeatedly ended up having special meaning for the Hight family.

I was born in a year ending in eight. Paul was fifteen years old and still in San Antonio at Saint John's at the time. My oldest brother might have been home at the time of my birth, along with Susan, John, Bill, and Marilyn, in that order—or maybe not. The Hight children seemingly came in three-year increments, as if Mom and Dad had planned an orderly cycle of birthing, which I can assure you was not the case.

On that Sunday, July 13, 1958, the Hights attended Sunday Mass at Saint Mary's as usual, followed by lunch at home. The dishes had barely been cleared from the table when Mom began to have labor pains. The contractions progressed into the evening and night hours until my parents finally decided that it was time to go to the hospital.

Dad rushed Mom to town—straight to the local Benedictine Heights Hospital for the impending birth of their fourth son and seventh child. Mom was in pain but calm and quiet as Dad drove. At the hospital, Dad led her up six flights of steps and inside. After six children, the place was familiar. All his children had been born there, including Paul, the future priest, on December 27, 1942, a Sunday, no less, when the place was still Cimarron Valley Wesley Hospital.

Paul Wilber Hight was most likely named after his mother and father. Pauline was thirty-eight and Wilber forty when I was born. I would learn the details of my birth during one of Dad and Uncle Lee's bull-shooting sessions. The oldest of Dad's brothers, Uncle Lee possessed a storytelling prowess that rivaled that of anyone in the Hight family. He and my Aunt Gladys no longer lived in Oklahoma; they were among the more than four hundred thousand Okies who had left the state during the Dust Bowl. In their case, they went in search of shipyard work in California. They were among the Hight children's favorite relatives. Uncle Lee and Dad, both with their prominent noses and strong but kind eyes, could sit for hours telling stories of their difficult childhoods growing up in Guthrie during the Great Depression. My dad was even known to turn over his rocking chair to Uncle Lee at times so my uncle could wax eloquent from the best spot in the living room.

One of Uncle Lee's best stories was about my birth. "I looked into the cradle and thought you were the biggest baby I'd ever seen in my life!" Uncle Lee would exclaim as he stretched out his hands to the size of a twenty-pound catfish. In reality, I weighed only about eight pounds at birth, but every time I heard the story, my birth weight grew until at some point I resembled a thirty-pound catfish, which would have meant I measured more than forty inches in length, taller than a toddler!

Dad would chime in: "Well, I couldn't get Pauline fast enough to the hospital when Joe was born. I swear we put Pauline on a gurney and rushed her into the elevator. When the elevator opened, there was Dr. Petty, but Joe had already been born! . . . I'm just glad I didn't drop him! He shot out like a circus performer from a cannon."

Uncle Lee's response to that was always, "He was the biggest baby I'd ever seen."

"And the fastest," Dad would reply, throwing his hands up in the air as if expecting another baby to fly out of that imaginary cannon.

Even though I was, according to the elder Hight brothers, apparently the fastest and biggest baby known to mankind, the seventh of seven children apparently didn't create the same photographic frenzy as the first born. Few photographs exist of me except for the annual school picture from Saint Mary's Catholic School, where I endured my fair share of hair pulling and ear tugging by the Benedictine nuns. I suspect Paul never had to endure any such indignities during his grade school years, although in fairness to my brother, that could have been due to his natural quiet and studious nature.

* * * * *

While still in seminary, Paul acquired a pale blue Volkswagen bug. The car fit Paul's personality, if not his long lanky body. The two-door Beetle was big enough, affordable enough, and simple—nothing fancy for my down-to-earth big brother. Paul drove the car back and forth from Saint Louis to Guthrie or to visit friends. The vehicle gave him a freedom he had never had and made it possible for him to avoid long bus rides or expensive plane flights, neither of which he particularly liked. That Beetle carried him everywhere until he wrecked the car on a trip to Guthrie for his ordination.

Paul's wrecked Volkswagen Mom wrote on photos showing the dented hood and disfigured passenger side of the car. Paul told friends the accident had scared him but it must have been God's will that he was spared injury right before his ordination and graduation. The little car was soon repaired, and Paul was back on the road again—only this time headed to a life in the priesthood.

Truth be told, growing up, I thought of Paul as a priest long before he became one. He was among only a few people whom I truly admired in life. To me, Paul was in the same league as Martin Luther King Jr., whom I admired for his pursuit of civil rights through nonviolence. I remember once asking my mother about my heritage, where I came from. Now if I had asked Dad that question, he might well have told me on one day that I was descended from the Cherokee tribe and the next day from Cole Younger and his outlaw band of brothers and on yet another day from Cole Younger's sister, who was a Cherokee princess. Mom was much more restrained in her response.

"Irish, English, Indian, German . . . you're a mix of about everything," she said.

"Even African?" I asked.

"Yes," she replied.

I can remember smiling at her answer, seeing in it proof that Martin Luther King was part of me and that I could share in his dream for this country too.

Thirteen days after the assassination of King and two months before Robert Kennedy's, in the midst of the Vietnam War, with the rise and beginning of the fall of Richard Nixon as a backdrop, Paul began his ascent to the priesthood. The national gloom that hung over the country would soon lift at home as we began to plan for Paul's ordination. It was April 1968. I was less than three months from my tenth birthday. And my parents' dream—our family's dream—for the nearly twenty-six-year-old Paul was finally becoming a reality.

We awaited his ordination ceremony with all the anticipation and excitement usually reserved for a big wedding to which the entire town would be invited. The boxes of cookies my mother had ordered for Paul's ordination reception began to fill our two-car garage. I remember sneaking into the garage and carefully opening one, two, maybe three or four of the boxes. The cookies were the kind that young boys dream about: shortbread, lemon cream, peanut butter, and so many other flavors. They were packed in square, vanilla-colored boxes and stacked four or five boxes high in the center of our garage. I would slither my fingers into a small opening in one, grab two to four cookies, tuck them under my shirt, and race to my bedroom for a cookie feast. The garage full of cookies was a symbol of the significance of Paul's ordination to a community such as Guthrie.

That process had started the previous May when the diocese sent to the Saint Louis seminary the "Form of Investigation and the Banns of Ordination for the Rev. Mr. Paul W. Hight who was promoted to the Sacred Orders of Subdeaconship and Deaconship at Kendrick last weekend." In the way the banns of marriage are announced publicly, so are the banns of ordination for future Catholic priests. The public announcement for Paul commanded a front-page article in the local *Guthrie Daily Leader* headlined "Bishop to Ordain Guthrian" that featured Paul's photo. The story was sandwiched among a story about the U.S.-Soviet race to land the first man on the moon, the police blotter, and the theft of a rabbit from its cage. That was likely the first time the Hights had been a page-one story since Linda's drowning in 1948. Thankfully, this time was for a happy occasion, but such are the things that nevertheless cross the mind, tingeing even the best of times with sadness. The story announced:

> The Rev. Mr. Paul Hight, son of Mr. and Mrs. Wilber Hight, east of Guthrie, will be ordained by Bishop Victor J. Reed at 7:30 p.m. Wednesday in Saint Mary's Catholic Church.

And the article went on to say that a reception would be held in the school gym immediately following the ceremony, and the public was invited to attend.

Just the fact that the ordination was being held in Guthrie was big news. Ordinations were usually held every other year at the Holy Family Cathedral in Tulsa or the Cathedral of Our Lady of Perpetual Help in Oklahoma City. However, Bishop Reed had begun to allow for an alternative location when the number of priests being ordained was small. One priest explained that most ordinations were on Saturdays at one of the two cathedrals, and some had been disorganized and not highly attended by other priests. The bishop hoped taking the ordinations to the hometowns would inspire other young men to become priests while also recognizing the seminarians' home parishes, the communities that had produced priests.

Fittingly, in the spirit of Vatican II, the entire town of Guthrie, Catholic or not, was invited to the reception.

* * * * *

At 7:30 p.m. April 17, 1968, on a cloudy, mild Oklahoma day the week after Easter Sunday, more than two dozen priests, a future bishop, and a current bishop joined a crowd of friends and family packed in the pews to witness a hometown boy's ordination. The church was Saint Mary's, which we had attended as a family for years, where priests were friends, where everyone knew your name.

Reed, the presiding bishop, was part of the five-man American liturgy commission responsible for implementing the mandates of the Second Vatican Council. Besides his progressive stance in the Catholic Church, Reed had spoken openly against the Vietnam War and for civil rights. He backed open housing for all races in Oklahoma City. A year before Paul's ordination, he had called for racial harmony in Oklahoma City, saying the city was close to "Detroit-type riots."

A polite and respectful leader who once said that he saw himself as "not easy to know, but I wear well," Reed sought to change the concept of the "ivory tower bishop," one who "would rather keep aloof above things . . . not fight it out." Such stances made him both beloved and vilified. He was known to spend hours praying in the chapel of his residence, the former Hales Mansion in downtown Oklahoma City, which also served as the chancery for the diocese.

A three-story, twenty-thousand-square-foot Renaissance Revival behemoth featuring imported Grecian brick, the home could accommodate a hundred people. Reed had converted an entryway on the second floor into a chapel. Built in 1916 by William T. Hales, a horse and mule trader, the mansion was purchased by the diocese with the help of Oklahoma oilman Frank Phillips after Hales's death. In 1985, Archbishop Charles Salatka, who came to Oklahoma from Marquette, Michigan, one of the country's poorest dioceses, had the mansion sold and the Archdiocesan offices moved to the former Saint Francis de Sales Seminary. The mansion sold for $1 million—bought by a family who made a $250,000 down payment and agreed to pay the remaining $750,000 over forty years at 8 percent interest, or $62,577 a year.

In 1968, however, the mansion still also served as a home for priests. One staff member remembered playing his drums in his room above the second floor where the bishop lived. Two years earlier, *Fortune* magazine had singled out Reed as heading "one of the most revolutionary Catholic communities in the United States," calling him the "local prophet of a new, more vital brand of Catholicism," according to *The Oklahoma Journal.* Many remember him as an intelligent man who respected those who opposed his views, even those who still wanted masses to be celebrated in Latin instead of English. He was also tolerant of protesters outside the mansion who opposed his antiwar sentiments.

Reed oversaw an ecumenical movement that allowed at least one Catholic parish to join the Greater Tulsa Council of Churches, as well as experiments in the liturgy, within prescribed limits. He began a movement to remove strict requirements that defrocked priests who married must "move to a place where their previous condition was unknown." One of his more controversial moves included reorganizing and renaming the diocesan newspaper to give it more freedom.

When *The Oklahoma Courier* began to criticize once sacred Catholic institutions and do in-depth stories on sensitive social issues such as racism, some nuns, priests, and laypeople questioned whether it should have the same First Amendment rights as secular newspapers.

At the time of Paul's ordination, Reed was also presiding over the intense proceedings by seven hundred delegates to the Oklahoma Little Council. The Little Council was considering issues in the Oklahoma City–Tulsa diocese such as communications, ecumenism, education, liturgy, parish structure, and social action. All were formulated by Reed to implement Vatican II in Oklahoma.

Only a month before Paul's ordination, Bishop Reed had said in an interview that although he appreciated the loyalty of his priests and certain people in the diocese, he was disappointed that the reforms of Vatican II had created such opposition and divisions.

"The impact has been considerably different than I had expected," he said. "I expected the people to be more receptive, not to have so much resistance as many have shown toward these changes in the Church. I felt that our people should have shown greater appreciation of human society, the need for the Church to change."

All of the turmoil caused by his newspaper and the changes he was making must have weighed on the bishop that April as he welcomed two more young men to the priesthood. Surely, the bishop's vow to "stand by his priests" had to give Paul confidence in what he was about to undertake.

Ordinations are long affairs, lasting as long as two hours, with a formal reception afterward. Clouds of incense fill the air during the ceremony, the scent permeating every nostril in attendance. The long procession, longer than any wedding ceremony, features altar servers, followed by a deacon carrying the Book of Gospels, the candidate for ordination, the priests who will concelebrate the Mass with the bishop and candidate, and finally the bishop between two deacons. The Knights of Columbus, with swords and regalia, are often in the procession too.

Our whole family attended Paul's ordination: Dad, Mom, Susan, John, Bill, Marilyn, and me, all in our finest clothing, which likely included a few pass-me-downs. John served as an altar boy and stood next to Paul during the ceremony. Our last living grandparent, Rosie Hight, whose landscapes still grace walls in Guthrie, was in the first row with us. Behind us were aunts, uncles, and cousins. The church was filled with members of the clergy, nuns, family friends, and fellow parishioners—women and girls in lace veils and dresses covering their knees, men in dark suits, white shirts, and narrow ties. Few would have dared to attend without first having donned the finest dress or suit they had.

Paul, however, wore a simple white vestment. His expression was serious, but his face glowed as if illuminated by sunshine as he processed with his parents beside him. The smirk that had characterized him in his early years was gone, replaced by a smile of serene confidence. His dark hair was cropped closely around his ears and slicked back with a hard part on the side. Only his black-rimmed glasses served as a reminder of his awkward teenage years.

Through my nine-year-old eyes, the ceremony seemed to entail Paul kneeling a lot and then spending a long spell facedown on the floor.

Much of the symbolism was lost on me. I didn't realize that in kneeling before Bishop Reed, Paul was pledging obedience to the bishop and his successors. I didn't understand that by lying prostrate on the floor, Paul was showing his unworthiness to serve in the priest's role and his dependence on God and the prayers of the community to be successful in his future ministry. Finally, in silence, the bishop and priests administered the laying on of the hands, the moment in which Paul officially entered the priesthood, one of the three ordained orders of the Catholic Church, along with bishop and deacon.

The prayer of consecration followed, and then Paul received his stole and chasuble, the outermost liturgical vestment worn by clergy when celebrating Mass. Together, the stole and chasuble signified the end of what had begun twelve years ago: the choices Paul had made—and those made for him to live away from home—finally had meaning.

* * * * *

The following Sunday, Father Paul Hight celebrated his first Mass at his childhood church in Guthrie on the feast of Saint Thomas, the apostle who refused to believe in the resurrected Jesus until he could see and feel the wounds Jesus suffered on the cross. Once again, the immediate Hight family was in attendance. Father John Sullivan, a family friend who later became a bishop serving in Nebraska and Missouri, gave the homily. After Mass, the family held another reception, in which the remainder of those tasty cookies from the ordination was served.

Looking back on that special day, I can't help but wonder if my parents' thoughts turned to the one member of our family who could not be physically with us—the little one for whom Father Sullivan had also celebrated a special Funeral Mass in this very same church so many years ago. If they did or if Paul's did, the rest of us children never knew it. There were only smiles that day—and Paul's solemn vow to serve the Roman Catholic Church and God and to follow in the footsteps of Christ in spreading the good news of the Bible, not in the Holy Land but on the prairie of Oklahoma to his fellow Oklahomans.

47

Yet possibly unbeknownst to him, Paul was entering uncertain times too. As Father James L. White, historian of the Diocese of Tulsa, wrote in *Tulsa: This Far by Faith 1875–2000*:

> Parish priests, who had received no seminary forma-
> tion in the issues under debate [post–Vatican II], were
> unprepared to introduce them to their congregations.
> And those responsible for scheduling the initial stages
> of reforms found themselves unable to provide guidance
> to a Catholic world that was increasingly confused and
> frightened by these difficult transitions.

How would my brother fare in a post–Vatican II world?

Chapter 6

The Role of the Priest

Paul was a natural priest. Among family and friends, he could be quiet and unassuming, fading at times into the background. In front of an audience or talking to someone about God, he became outgoing and confident—his voice boomed and his smile broadened. He acquired a deep belly laugh that could fill a crowded room.

After returning to Saint Louis to graduate from the seminary, Paul was assigned to the Tulsa region of the Oklahoma City–Tulsa Diocese. He would later write that his specific duties included "preaching, leader of church services, visitation of sick and elderly, supervised religious instruction," and "help charitable activities." His choice of the word *preaching* instead of *giving homilies*, the usual Catholic term for sermons, may have stemmed from his desire to both introduce people to the Lord and encourage them to follow in the footsteps of Jesus on a daily basis as well as his father's lingering Baptist influence.

Paul's instincts were in keeping with the spirit of Vatican II, which hoped to instill a more pastoral focus in the Church, with priests focusing less on religiosity and more on helping people live the faith in their daily lives.

Paul believed the priesthood was a calling, a lifetime vocation, not a job that one could quit. The Catholic Church had long seen it that way as well, as Psalm 110:4 says:

> Yahweh has sworn an oath he will never retract, you
> are a priest forever . . .

The Catholic catechism states that the sacrament of Holy Orders confirms an "indelible spiritual character" on the man who receives it, and, as with the sacrament of Baptism, one that can never be erased . . . once a priest, always a priest.

Oh, if that were only true.

But that sorrow for Paul was yet to come.

For his first priestly assignment, Paul was sent far from his home parish, where he had been ordained and had said his first Mass. Such was the case for most new priests, and it meant Paul was starting his new life far away from the influence of his family and friends. Paul's parish family was to be his new family, as the Church believed it should be. Fellow priests were his new brotherhood. He belonged to God, the Catholic Church, the bishop, and his pastor and congregation in that order. Only then did his biological family come into play.

He was assigned as an assistant to Father Philip Bryce at Saint John the Evangelist Catholic Church in McAlester, Oklahoma. The city of nearly nineteen thousand nestled in the hills of rural southeastern Oklahoma is best known for the Oklahoma State Penitentiary, home to the state's most hardened criminals and death row. McAlester was a stark change from Paul's hometown of Guthrie, which, although half the size, sat on the busy north-south artery of Interstate 35, thirty minutes north of the Oklahoma City metro area.

Paul was succeeding two assistant pastors at a parish rich with history. Twelve priests first traveled to what would become McAlester with Spanish explorer Hernando de Soto on an expedition in 1541. Another three hundred years would pass before missionaries returned in 1847 and nearly a half century more before construction started on Saint

John's in 1895. Still, that was more than a decade before Oklahoma became a state in 1907.

The parish included the church, a school with two hundred students run by Benedictine nuns, and missions in Eufaula, McIntosh County, and the local state prison. A week after his arrival, Paul was featured in a page-two story in the *McAlester News-Capital* on Tuesday, June 18:

> A vibrant new voice was heard this past week by the parishioners of Saint John's Catholic Church.
>
> The voice was that of Rev. Paul Hight, the impressive young priest who has arrived to take on the duties of assistant pastor.
>
> Newly ordained . . . Rev. Hight seems to vibrate the young and fresh look of the Church today, and readily admits his endorsement of the changes.
>
> "Most resent the changing of the beautiful old traditions which are basically European," he explained. "However, the American Church is coming to age now, and will be just as beautiful as what it replaced."
>
> . . . Rev. Hight expressed his delight that his first assignment is McAlester explaining that it is considered one of the best assignments in the diocese because of it's [sic] challenge.
>
> "It has a great variety of work," he said, "because of the state prison and the Eufaula mission."

Prison ministry was exactly the kind of social justice outreach that Vatican II reforms were meant to encourage in Catholics, and Paul took to it. Before long, he was not only visiting inmates but also referring to some of them as friends. "He liked the people in prison. He thought all of them were great guys," said Bill Hight, who had visited Paul in McAlester. A decade younger than Paul and the second youngest of the Hights' four sons, Bill watched, a little aghast, as Paul downplayed the danger some of his new friends might present.

To Paul, the difference between good and bad was minute, and Bill feared that left his brother open to being conned or even hurt. More than once, Bill tried to tell his older brother that the inmates at the state prison were there because they had committed serious crimes: murder, assault, robbery, and rape. Many were hardened criminals, some serving life sentences or even awaiting execution.

"He had a misconception about the difference between someone who was bad and someone who would con you," Bill said. "He saw the good in individuals no matter how bad they were. He didn't know the difference between someone conning him and someone truly in need."

Meanwhile, although his local parish duties kept him busy on a daily basis, Paul remained interested in the issues of the larger Catholic Church, a Church grappling with change.

On July 25, 1968, Pope Paul VI rejected the theological findings of his own Papal Birth Commission when he issued the papal encyclical *Humanae vitae*, or "Of Human Life," which upheld the Church's 1930 ban on the use of artificial contraception.

The pope wrote that parents:

> . . . are not free to proceed completely at will, as if they could determine in a wholly autonomous way the honest path to follow; but they must conform their activity to the creative intention of God, expressed in the very nature of marriage and of its acts, and manifested by the constant teaching of the Church.

Another section in Pope Paul VI's letter directly addressed priests:

> Your first task . . . is to expound the Church's teaching on marriage without ambiguity. Be the first to give, in the exercise of your ministry, the example of loyal internal and external obedience to the teaching authority of the Church.

The papal letter created turmoil inside and outside the Catholic Church—eventually six hundred Catholic theologians, including some priests, in the United States signed on to a statement of dissent.

The progressive Oklahoma diocese was especially turbulent. In mid-August 1968, the College of Oklahoma Priests issued a statement opposing the Pope's encyclical and stating that married couples should ultimately make their own decisions on contraception. Of the 213 priests in Oklahoma counted as considering the statement, seventy-two signed it, thirty-one declined to endorse it, and 110 did not respond either way. Paul Hight was among the seventy-two Oklahoma priests who signed the statement, which read:

> The recently published encyclical *Humanae Vitae* of Paul VI expresses many positive values concerning marriage, including its emphasis upon the need for a total vision of man and the importance of conjugal love and responsible parenthood in all aspects of the relationship between husbands and wives. We may neither disregard the pope's teachings nor fail to make every effort to be understanding of the grave reasons that led him to issue this document. However, we also respectfully recognize that the encyclical, although authentic (i.e., truly reflecting the mind of the pope), is not an infallible teaching (i.e., irrevocable and demanding a total assent of faith). The encyclical may not be disregarded, and certainly the pope's statement introduces an important new element—his own authoritative judgment of the issues involved . . .
>
> Catholic theology has always taught that a grave obligation may never be imposed upon the Christian conscience unless the obligation itself is absolutely certain, and the pope's encyclical has not decisively altered the situation of practical doubt which existed within the Church prior to its publication.

Therefore, any Catholic couple seeking to form their own conscience regarding contraception should seriously take into consideration the encyclical inasmuch as it is an authoritative statement, but they also have a right and duty to arrive at a responsible decision concerning this matter on their own case. Should they conscientiously decide, before God, that artificial contraception is permissible and indeed necessary in certain circumstances in order to preserve and foster their values and sacredness of their marriage, they should still consider themselves Catholics in good standing.

As pastors and confessors, we recognize that it is our responsibility to aid couples in understanding the importance of the issues involved, but we cannot appropriate ourselves a decision which is rightfully theirs to make.

Many of those who signed the statement were pastors and Church leaders; some eventually left the priesthood but many remained priests for the rest of their lives. How difficult would it have been for a priest who had been ordained for less than six months to step up and sign such a statement? Paul might have been the newest priest to do so.

With Bishop Reed still leading the diocese, Oklahoma priests, including the newest one, at least had more latitude. They could openly oppose a pope's encyclical, maybe even go as far as Paul did to sign and declare it not an infallible document. Other priests in other parts of the country had no such freedom. Cardinal Patrick O'Boyle, who had set about desegregating Catholic schools in the Washington, D.C., area before the 1954 *Brown v. Board of Education* decision, this time gave the fifty-one signers among his 385 priests an ultimatum: Either recant opposition to the pope's letter, what he called "an attack on authority," or face penalties.

That was not how things unfolded in Oklahoma. Paul's reasons for signing the document might have come from his own insecurities when it came to counseling couples about marriage. During a dinner with family, he once asked, "What do I know about a relationship between a man and woman?" That was a question for which even the Hights had no answer, but as with so many Catholics, the Church would be their ultimate guide.

* * * * *

In 1969, Paul was transferred to a new parish. This time, he returned to a metropolitan area, but one where he had never been: Tulsa, in the northeastern part of the state.

For a short time, he was assigned to Holy Family Cathedral, where he was given a spartan room not much larger than a dorm room or a monastery cell. The room had a dark wood floor, and furnishings consisted of a simple twin bed with a lamp beside it, a small desk with a chair, a statue of Mary on the desk, and a simple cross nailed to the wall—exactly what Paul wanted in a home.

His first duty was also what my brother wanted and might well have been his favorite assignment as a priest: He was named the liaison to Catholic parishes fighting for social justice and against poverty in Tulsa.

"[Paul] was very devoted to the poor. He had such a good heart," recalled Father Lowell Stieferman, another humble Oklahoma priest, in an interview before his death in 2016. Father Martin Morgan also remembered Paul taking on the assignment as his "own personal responsibility, especially in how he worked with the poor." A Scranton, Pennsylvania, native who became a seminarian in Ardmore and was ordained there two years later, in 1970, Morgan remained in Oklahoma and now is in the Tulsa Diocese.

Paul would work with three Tulsa parishes: Saint Jude's under Father Dan Allen, Saint Monica's under Father Forrest "Babe" O'Brien, and Immaculate Conception under Father Lee O'Neil. Allen's efforts to put faith into action resulted in the formation of Neighbor for Neighbor, which to this day offers programs to assist the uninsured, low-income, unemployed, elderly, handicapped, and impoverished in Tulsa.

The assignment would impact Paul as a priest and personally for the rest of his life. But first, it would place him in the middle of mounting tensions between the more affluent south side of Tulsa and the poorer north side, as that trio of priests began to challenge the status quo as it pertained to economic inequality in the community. "Priests who embraced the cause of social activism frequently expressed contempt for Catholics who live middle-class lives," Jeremy Bonner wrote about the three priests in *The Road to Renewal: Victor Joseph Reed and Oklahoma Catholicism, 1905–1971*.

Another prominent Catholic in the diocese would say years later that all three of the priests Paul worked with thought, "Rich is a sin. Poor is a virtue. They thought the priesthood should be a democracy. They were very serious but had little humor. You were for them or against them." He saw their work not as doing God's work but as a rebellion against the Tulsa elite, a rebellion bolstered by the priests and laypeople whom they recruited to their cause. Bonner recalls a dinner at which Catholic lay leader and attorney Douglas Fox, who served on Reed's finance committee, attempted to forge a better rapport with Allen, O'Brien, and O'Neil. However, the three priests quickly denounced south Tulsans, including Fox, as being indifferent to human suffering and the plight of the poor and largely black population on the city's north side. "Some of you will at least write checks, but that's all you ever want to do," Allen told Fox. Although Fox is my wife's uncle, I would only learn about the dinner in the course of my research; he did confirm the dinner occurred.

The brouhaha over the three priests became so intense at one point that a wealthy Tulsan told Bishop Reed that if he were bishop, he would have fired the three over their actions. Reed's reply: "They don't work for me. They work for the Church." Once again, Reed's steadfast support of his priests did not waver, even for those who created turmoil for him.

As time passed, Allen became more outspoken about issues involving poverty and civil rights in Tulsa. In an interview for CBS News about Neighbor for Neighbor, Allen contended that south Tulsa was built by the poor of north Tulsa. "The facade is beautiful, but the guts— the guts are full of cancer," Allen said in the interview. The "Church was useless if it would not take its stand with the defenseless." Allen would also become friends with Father Bill Skeehan, another antipoverty crusader on behalf of north Tulsans. When Allen became pastor of Saint Jude's Catholic Church in 1966, he turned the church grounds, including the parking lot, into donation sites, places where those who had too much could share what they had with those who had so little.

Eventually, Allen turned his rectory into an incubator for social justice. Neighbor for Neighbor came from the discussions and exchange of ideas that went on there, as did his and Skeehan's "Give a Damn" campaign to fight poverty in north Tulsa. As a history of the Dan Allen Center for Social Justice would later admit, Allen's efforts were "ramshackle, untidy, and endlessly creative." Yet all these years later, the Dan Allen Center still exists, collaborating with the Tulsa City-County Library and holding an annual awards program to encourage those who work for social justice in the Tulsa community. Allen went on to leave the priesthood to devote his energy full time to Neighbor for Neighbor until his death at age sixty-five in 1995.

From his work with such priests, Paul developed a black-and-white sense of right and wrong as well as a soft heart for the poor. Father Morgan, who had known Paul from priest gatherings and dinners, said years later, "[Paul] had an exacting sense of right and wrong. He was intensely spiritual. He was not a preachy person. He was always trying to be more of a ministerial person. He led with his service."

Paul's meager monthly salary of about $125 usually went not to his wants and needs but to anyone he met in need. He was highly protective of the poor box and special collections for the poor, wanting to ensure that every nickel went to the less fortunate. At one point, he told both a priest and his family his suspicion that certain priests were dividing funds from the poor box and special collections among themselves or using them for other than their intended purposes. He eventually took his concerns to a higher authority but was reportedly reprimanded for questioning the actions and motives of his fellow priests.

As so often happens with whistle-blowers, Paul's actions drew not appreciation but resentment, and they distanced him from certain priests in the diocese. Like an honest cop in a corrupt precinct, his efforts were used against him to fuel doubt about Paul's dedication to the brotherhood.

Certain priests—especially those who drank heavily, cursed openly, and told off-color stories—resented the young priest questioning their actions and motives. Some of Paul's harshest critics were the older priests who had come to Oklahoma decades before from Ireland. Despite his own Irish ancestry, Paul, like his own Irish-American mother, rarely cursed or drank alcohol. Paul believed a priest should behave in private as he would in public, as these very same priests told their parishioners they should behave. Ironically, the response of the older priests was to tell Paul to quit being so self-righteous.

Meanwhile, in the Catholic Church, the times were a-changin', as Bob Dylan wrote in 1964, and Vatican II was only partly the reason. Priests were leaving the Church in alarming numbers—and not in protest over Vatican II. The Religious News Service reported that one priest quit every day from 1966 to 1967, with many people at the time convinced that the numbers understated the problem. RNS research indicated a trend on the upswing, a view supported by news service findings that forty-three U.S. dioceses and 135 of 160 male religious communities had not even bothered to report the priests who had departed.

In the age of free love, most priests who left the priesthood did so to marry, with some apparently doing so to test the Church's celibacy requirements. That can be seen in the 1963 ordination class in Oklahoma, a state by no means a bailiwick of Catholicism when compared with, say, New York or Illinois or Pennsylvania. Yet by the time Paul had been reassigned to Tulsa in 1969, five of the eleven men in the 1963 class had left the priesthood. Bishop Reed saw his administrative staff dwindle to two because of the defections. One of those who left married a nun. The leavings became so frequent that priests joked that if a certain priest hadn't shown up for dinner yet, he had left the priesthood.

Possibly the most notable Oklahoma defection was William "Bill" Garthoeffner, who had been Bishop Reed's chancellor. *Road to Renewal* describes Garthoeffner as Reed's alter ego, a priest who became one of the bishop's leading spokesmen on Vatican II reforms and was named episcopal vicar of Oklahoma's western district. The admiration was mutual. Reed believed in the younger priest and promoted him thusly, and Garthoeffner believed in Bishop Reed, years later calling him a positive, intelligent, holy man always concerned about his priests. Reed was a bishop whose efforts in pushing the reforms of Vatican II, Garthoeffner believed, were also appreciated by most of his priests, many of whom were excited about the spirit of change swirling through the Church. Nonetheless, Garthoeffner left the priesthood, in his case, to marry. "[Bishop Reed] was disappointed when I left the priesthood," said Garthoeffner, his voice crackling with age and lowering in sadness at the memory. "He considered me a friend."

By the early Seventies, Bill Garthoeffner and Tulsa antipoverty crusader Father "Babe" O'Brien were among an estimated 30 percent of American priests who had left the priesthood. ABC News would later report, "Although there are several factors, the Church's celibacy rule is widely considered the major cause of an exodus of priests in the 1960s and 1970s, and is cited as the No. 1 reason young men leave seminaries before they are ordained."

Father Stieferman was among those who believed many of the former priests had made hasty decisions. "Most of the marriages didn't work," he said. "Many messed up their lives."

The exodus, however, created voids and shortages in parishes, and many young and older priests were thrust into positions with more responsibility than would normally have been the case. Paul was one such priest for which this was true. He was moved from his liaison position to be associate pastor of Saints Peter and Paul in northeast Tulsa. The other associate at the parish was Father Stieferman, and Stieferman remembered Paul being disappointed about being pulled so quickly from the antipoverty team in Tulsa.

Soon, Paul was in the parish Mass rotation, a rotation structured so that parishioners would never know which priest would be presiding over which Mass. The system was a way of keeping parishioners from favoring one priest over another.

Paul developed an easygoing homily style, often stepping out from behind the pulpit and away from his notes so that nothing separated him from the congregation. He relayed stories and shared personal experiences along with the prescribed Bible passages specified by the liturgical calendar. He talked about Jesus and how his death saved humans from sin, not unlike an evangelical minister. He used his booming voice to provide emphasis, but he also spoke slowly and softly at times, deliberately choosing words and details to paint a better picture and induce a clearer understanding of the Good Word. "It was very easy to listen to his sermons," a person who attended several of Paul's masses once said. "You would be listening for fifteen to twenty minutes, and soon the sermon would be over, and you'd say to yourself, 'I want more.' "

In keeping with the post–Vatican II times, Paul often sang and played his guitar at youth masses, nursing homes, and youth group gatherings, his deep voice bellowing sweet, low notes to the twangs of his guitar. After Mass, he didn't linger, instead walking straight outside so he could visit with as many people as possible, smiling broadly at each person while shaking hands and giving hugs. Even with the parish's secret rotation, his masses were usually filled, and parishioners weren't above calling the parish office to ask when Paul would be saying Mass that weekend. In the aftermath of Vatican II, a Saturday evening Mass had been added that fulfilled the Sunday Mass obligation.

This was a happy period in my brother's life and priesthood. No one remembers any signs of mental illness—not family, not friends, not his fellow priests, not even our cousin, Arlene Meier, who worked as a nurse in a psychiatric hospital. Paul kept his personal issues private, and of the people he confided in then, what most of them remembered was that Paul's concerns centered on his insecurities as a priest, his worry that he was not doing all he could for his flock.

Arlene, however, had witnessed firsthand the deep sadness in the Hight house in the days following Linda's death all those years ago, because her mother, our father's sister, had decided Arlene's cheerful personality was needed there during that difficult time. Arlene still remembered her visit vividly, especially her Uncle Wilber telling her that losing Linda was the worst sorrow he had ever felt. Arlene worried that losing his little sister might still haunt Paul.

Occasionally, after he became a priest, Paul would visit Arlene's folks for dinner. Uncle Kenneth and Aunt Lillian McWethy's home was always open to any of the Hight children, and Aunt Lillian was a trusted counselor to Paul. She might have been why Paul was open to other religions because, unlike her brother, Aunt Lillian was still a practicing Protestant. Paul and Aunt Lillian talked openly and vigorously about their faith, their respective denominations, and issues without becoming judgmental of each other. Arlene remembers her mother sometimes asking Paul to say the prayer before dinner. At the Hights and at most Catholic tables, that would be:

> Bless us, Oh Lord, and these thy gifts, which we are about to receive, from thy bounty, through Christ, Our Lord. Amen.

Certain family members might say the prayer faster than others, especially if Mom's fried chicken was being served, but that was the standard dinner prayer at the Hights'. But on this evening, Arlene remembered thinking Paul seemed more confident than in the past. He still seemed his usual quiet and gentle self, at least until he began to pray.

"He became fairly loud," Arlene said. "He recited the words as if he were reciting the words from *Are You Running with Me, Jesus*. It wasn't the prescribed [Catholic] prayer."

In a booming voice, Paul prayed:

> Run with me, Jesus! Run with us today. Thank you, Jesus!

And Arlene's instincts were right. The words were a paraphrase of *Are You Running with Me, Jesus*, the best-selling book of prayers published in 1965 by the late Episcopal priest and author Malcolm Boyd, who encouraged people to pray in more conversational tones as if Jesus were a friend. Boyd was said to have taken prayer out of the church onto the city streets.

At another family dinner with the McWethys, Paul talked about his own belief in the power of prayer, sharing a story of a young blind teenager he had met while visiting her family in rural Guthrie. The girl's parents had invited Paul to visit them, and during his visit, they asked him to pray for their daughter. Paul said he diligently prayed for the girl and took to visiting her when he was in the area. He encouraged others to do the same. The girl soon regained her vision. "God restored her vision because of our prayers," Paul told the McWethys that evening.

Nearly fifty years later, Arlene recalled, "[Paul] really believed that if he prayed hard enough that God would intervene."

Yet prayer could not save his own Grandma Hight. Eighty-four years old and a lifelong chain smoker, Grandma had skin that was leathery from smoking and hands yellowed from cigarette stains. Her time had come. However, Paul made it clear that he thought prayer would heal her.

"When Grandma Hight died, it was real upsetting to him," Arlene remembered. "He had been praying for her, and she died anyway."

Still, neither the turmoil at his parish nor the failure of some prayers lessened his faith or deterred his commitment to share the Word with others, especially children. I remember him returning to Saint Mary's to say Mass for my school, which sat next door to the church. Accustomed to the little slaps and frowns the nuns used to keep us quiet in the pews during the priest's homily, we were a little unsettled to have Paul grin as he began his. He didn't lecture us as the priest normally did. Instead, he strolled to the front of the sanctuary and began to ask questions:

"Do you know who Jesus is?"

"Do you know what he did that is so important to our lives today?"

"How can we live like Jesus?"

"How can we help the poor like Jesus did?"

If Paul expected an answer or a reaction, I'm afraid we failed him. We just sat stunned. It was unheard of for a priest to strike up a conversation in the middle of Mass. Some of us stole glances at each other as if a spotlight had been suddenly shone on us. And a few hands shot up in the air. The questions and answers went on for a few minutes as a full-fledged conversation ensued, one in which we listened and learned and participated instead of sitting like rows of stones as we usually did, fearful that our slightest move might draw an ear tug from a nun. As we walked back to school that day, my classmates could be heard chirping that it was the best Mass they had ever witnessed. My hero, my oldest brother, had come through again. I arrived home that afternoon and breathlessly told my mother the whole story. My preteen vocabulary struggled to convey the magnitude of what had taken place.

"Mama, he was asking us questions, and we were answering. We were laughing at some of things he was telling us," I said, searching for a word like *awesome* that didn't yet exist in that context. "I want to be like him, Mama! I want to be a priest."

My mother looked at me with her soft eyes and, still smiling, shook her head. "Joe, you can be anything you want in life. I just don't think being a priest would fit you. One priest in our family is already enough."

She fixed me a peanut-butter-and-jelly sandwich and, I assume, figured I'd forget about my newfound aspiration. I have often wondered about her motivation that day. Did she fear sending another son, her youngest son, away to seminary at age fourteen? Did she truly believe the role of priest would never suit me? Or did she see the strain of Paul trying to be the perfect priest and want to spare me such pressure and pain?

In the Catholic Church, a condition known as scrupulosity, or religious OCD, dates to the 1600s, when monks were found to be engaging in excessive prayer in an effort to achieve a perfect state of holiness. In modern times, the condition might manifest itself in a priest as a constant worry or regret about the smallest of perceived infractions—a too sharp glance, an abrupt response, a stray unholy thought, basically the fear of doing something, anything, in any given moment that doesn't align with one's idea of perfect behavior. For a priest who believes he is a living image of Jesus Christ, such fears can become debilitating.

Could my brother have begun to succumb to an impossible idea of the priesthood he could never achieve? If so he would not be the first. Father David Monahan, the beloved founding editor of *The Sooner Catholic* newspaper in Oklahoma City, was open about his own struggle to overcome the sin of scrupulosity. In fact, he always said it was one of his greatest personal struggles and admitted that the pressure to never misstep wore on this down-to-earth, funny priest like few could imagine, except for maybe his spiritual adviser.

Whatever Mom's impression was of her oldest son, my impression about Paul as a child was affirmed: He was my hero. He was perfect in my young eyes. But what about Paul's self-image? What about the regrets he still carried from his supposed role in the loss of his little sister all those years ago and his father's implication that he was to blame?

Time would not heal this gentle man.

Chapter 7

The Dream of Heaven and Hell

The call came early one morning in the summer of 1970 before the sun had roared into the sky and turned the heat blistering. I was still a child at home, and I awoke to the sound of my father talking loudly on the phone in a flustered tone.

A priest at Saints Peter and Paul Church was telling him that Paul was in jail. The police had found my brother wandering the streets near the rectory late the previous night. When stopped, Paul had told the officers he was "doing the work of God" and to leave him alone. When questioned further, he became belligerent and refused to give his name, so the police had taken him into custody.

"We'll be there as soon as possible," Dad told the priest.

Writing this, I can't help but think of that first assignment of Paul's that took him across the state from his family, in part to help him reshuffle the priorities of his life: God, the Catholic Church, the bishop, his pastor, his fellow priests, and his congregation. He belonged to them. Where were they now in his time of need?

That question would come to haunt me as an adult. But at the time of the phone call, I was barely out of sixth grade, the only nonteenager left in the Hight household. My brothers and sisters had either moved out to start their own adult lives or were in high school or away at college. My parents had entered their fifties, and my father had begun to talk retirement. Coworkers were dropping dead on the job from stress at the Air Logistics Center, he said, and he didn't want to do the same. The family garden was smaller than it had ever been, and I was selling what I could out of it to make some extra money. Mom had started talking about taking a dream trip to Hawaii, and I had promised I would earn enough to take her to the Big Island someday. She had also begun to hope for grandchildren. Both Dad and Mom considered Paul settled and doing well as an associate pastor, although they might have secretly hoped he would be made a pastor someday soon.

That call changed all of that.

What followed was in some ways more brutal than the day they lost Linda. As quickly as possible, Dad, Mom, and I climbed into the family Chevrolet Impala and drove to Tulsa, about a two-hour drive. As was customary in the Hight family when dealing with bad news, little was said during the trip. I crawled into the back seat and tried to sleep. Always a light sleeper, I was awakened by the sound of my mother's voice.

"Why?" she asked. She was speaking to my father. Dad only shook his head. My mother did not ask again. She turned her eyes to the ribbon of road ahead of us, staring into the early morning darkness. I fell asleep to the sound of her sniffling.

"Get up, Joe! We're here." My father's stern command brought me out of my slumber. I crawled from the car and walked with my parents to the front door of the rectory. Before Dad could knock, the door creaked open, revealing the dark shadow of a man who appeared to be a priest. My mother grabbed me by the arm and motioned for me to stay with her; we stepped back about ten feet. In a hushed tone, the man began to tell Dad what he knew about Paul's arrest. I glanced at Mom and noticed that stress wrinkles had spread across her face like a spider's web.

Every so often, Dad would say, "What?" in an unbelieving tone. The hushed voice would respond in a reassuring voice. Dad would calm down, and the conversation would continue. When everything that needed to be said right then had been said, Dad took his leave, signaling for us to return to the car. "We're going to pick up Paul and bring him back to the rectory. There must be some kind of explanation," he said.

"Do you know any more about what happened?" Mom asked quietly in a pleading voice I didn't recall her ever having used before.

"A little, but not enough to understand. Paul will have to explain."

"Well, there must be a good reason," Mom said. "This is so strange."

Then, silence again. The atmosphere was so tense that I dared not speak. It reminded me of the time I fell asleep only to wake minutes before I needed to be at school for a basketball game—and had the audacity to yell at my mother for making me late.

"Why didn't you wake me up?" I yelled.

The words had barely cleared my mouth before I felt the backside of my father's hand against my face. The force landed me, stunned but in one piece, against the dining room wall. As enraged as my mother surely was with me that day, she responded to my father's slap with the most seething glare I had ever seen from her. After making sure I was okay and telling me to go get ready for the game, she stormed into their bedroom, slamming the door behind her. Dad followed, and I will never forget the scream that came next:

"Never, ever touch a child of mine again! Or I'll . . ."

"But, Pauline, he . . ."

Mom was the one who drove me to the basketball game that afternoon. I never yelled at my mother again and my father never laid another hand on me. Unsure if this time would end so well, quiet I remained. I must have fallen asleep again too, because the next thing I remember is seeing Dad and Paul out the car window. Dad looked exasperated and Paul emotionless. "Okay, this can wait until after we're back at the rectory," Dad finally said.

Paul, ever the good soldier, shook his head in resignation and climbed into the car.

"Joe, straighten up and let Paul in," Dad ordered.

I quickly obeyed. Mom looked at Paul, her eyes full of disappointment and worry. Paul didn't respond. I dozed off, resorting to my usual coping mechanism on this difficult day. I didn't wake up until we were back at the rectory, and only then at my mother's urging. Paul led us down a dark hallway to a living room that reminded me of a funeral parlor, only larger. My father told me to take a seat on the couch, while he talked with Paul in the bedroom. Upon their return, Mom sent me to an adjoining room. I did as I was told, but if they were trying to shield me, they failed miserably. As I hid behind a wall, I overheard everything said. The words and images Paul revealed that day seemed biblical. This is the story my brother told as I remember it:

As I laid down on my bed last night. I found I was in a state of being awake while I was in the state of sleep. I couldn't move my body, but I was fully awake. Satan suddenly appeared in my room. He told me that I was meddling too much in the priests' affairs, and that I shouldn't be so judgmental about what they did with the collections. "You don't get paid that much, now do you?" Satan said. "Well, they get paid the same amount, hardly enough to live a decent life outside this rectory. It's not bad to want things for yourself—things that the Church would never let you have. There's so much that you can have if you follow me."

The devil commanded my spirit to follow him, and I could do nothing to resist as together we rose above the bed. I looked down and saw my body laying prostrate, face up on the twin bed below. I had been so tired I'd left my collar on. My glasses were on the nightstand. I laughed as I heard soft, snoring sounds coming from my mouth. I felt no pain even as I strained to see my body below. Satan told me to follow him to "my home—one that could be your home forever."

We descended quickly through the ground to the top of a mountain where Satan guided me to the highest point. I could see people below who were laughing while feasting on a large meal. Fire was not burning at their heels as I had thought there would be in hell. Satan motioned with his hand toward the valley.

"Paul, you could join my people who are sinners just like you, but they were redeemed by me and sent to this lovely place of places because they gave their hearts and souls to me. They love me. If you devote yourself to me, love me before any other god, I will save you from death—and fire." Satan then motioned beyond the valley. As he did, I could suddenly hear muttering, groaning, and wailing from a mass wave of dark shadows. Flames that gave off no smoke flickered above their shadowy figures—the size of the group seemed much larger than the joyous ones I had just seen.

"You have a choice: Follow me and be a leader in the valley of peace or continue to question my ways, continue to lead people away from me, continue to argue with those who seek greater means for themselves, then you will be cast in the dark shadow of shame and flames and loathing, always to burn, always to regret. Now what say you?"

When I shook my head no, the devil grabbed me and thrust me back into my room in the rectory. As we hovered above my prone body, Satan repeated "What say you?"

"No!" I said. "Your way is not my way. Go! Leave me alone. A false god shall never tempt me. Never!"

Like a salesman making a last-ditch pitch, Satan repeated his offer once more: "Live and lead in the valley of peace. The place you've always wanted. The place that you've denied yourself all these years. No hunger. No guilt. No pain. Just love of me and yourself, and peace with others like you."

"Do not tempt me, Satan!" I said.

Then, as quickly as he had arrived, Satan left, giving one last warning: "The voices of hell will always be with you the rest of your earthly life. You will never, ever know peace again. This is your fate—forever. You will be sorry."

A few minutes later, an angel came to me, fluttering again above. He was larger than Satan, with gentle eyes and a soft face that seemed to glow. "I am God's chosen one to show you the true way," the angel said.

Once more, my spirit rose high above my bed, and as I looked down, I saw my prone body had turned over in bed with arms outstretched as if reaching for something just out of reach. Again, I heard soft snoring coming from my mouth. "Yes, I will go where you want," I told the angel.

We ascended through the ceiling into a starry night sky, tinted by occasional cumulus clouds majestically anticipating an approaching storm. We soared above the clouds and stopped short of a large gate, which seemed to hover just above the clouds with a bright light shining on it.

"Satan was giving you an illusion of 'his' world. It is actually dark shadows of those who have turned away from the one and only true God, and who are now wailing in their own shame and grief, and toiling under the whips and chains of Satan's evil angels. Here, you will see the way toward the light in which you will be among the kings and queens of the enlightened—those who have not turned away, who have not been swayed by Satan's false words. This is the place in which you will see those who have truly been enlightened by God's wisdom and love and have followed the only way."

As I looked toward the gate of what I thought was heaven, my eyes cleared of their nearsightedness and the astigmatism I've had since childhood. I saw the gate opening softly without the creaking moans of the gate I had seen with Satan. In the distance, a man who looked like Jesus Christ walked toward me along with a woman who appeared to be in her early thirties wearing a jeweled crown of rubies and diamonds. Her eyes twinkled with happiness as she turned to the man, who stopped and motioned the woman toward me. Instantly, I knew who she was. "Linda, you're all grown up. I thought . . . thought I would never see you again."

"Yes, it's me, Paul! Here, we are all the same—never too young, never too old. I know you have been through much in your life. But persevere, Paul, persevere. You are leading the life that God has set before you. The life that will eventually lead you to this place of joy, no suffering, no ridicule, no deceit. Never forget that I am here, waiting for you."

She stepped back, and the man stepped forward. "I am who you think I am: the son of God. Like me, you will suffer great pain in your earthly life. You will die at the hands of people in authority who you do not know. But remember, your life will not be in vain if you continue in your path toward me." With no further words, the man turned and walked with Linda toward the pearly gate, but just before they entered, Linda turned around, looked gently back at me, and smiled. I understood that she was truly happy.

Before I could think another thought, the angel took my arm, and we descended back into my room in the rectory. As we hovered over my bed, the angel said: "Voices of evil will haunt you the remainder of your life, but they someday will be your salvation."

At that point, I was thrust back into my body. I woke, soaked with sweat, and searched for any signs that my vivid dream had happened. Then a voice in my head said: "Leave this evil place! Leave!" I ran from the room as the voice demanded: "Tell no one who you are, for they are after you to do you harm."

"Who?" I asked.

"Do not question me! Leave! The only safety is outside. Do not return until I tell you."

So, I left, and a couple of hours later, the police approached me. The voice continued to tell me not to say anything to the officers. And so I didn't.

My brother's words as spoken had chilled me as I listened to his story. The idea of Paul descending into hell and ascending into heaven seemed outlandish, but for a twelve-year-old reared in a devout Catholic home, who had gone to a Catholic school and studied the Bible and the lives of the saints, it did not seem impossible. Paul's visions sounded both real and terrifying. I became immersed in the story, so much so that I would remember his words for the rest of my life and eventually write down the full story of Paul's dream.

Despite all that had happened, Paul managed to convince Mom and Dad that he was fine. Reluctantly, my parents left. Paul stood outside, waving as we drove away. I waved back; my parents did not. They sat stone-faced as if they had just left a family member's funeral.

It would be years before I realized what they must have been thinking on that long drive home: Their handsome oldest son with the voice, the command, and the personality to go far in the Church was gone. In a single night, all their dreams for Paul had been taken away.

As for me, the story Paul had told had seemed real, but even I knew that it would be off-putting for most people, especially those closest to him. I realized the sunny dream of Paul as the perfect priest was gone for my parents, replaced by a dark shadow over what his future might now hold.

They could not begin to imagine what was to come.

Chapter 8

Something Is Wrong with Father

Our family soon learned that Paul's encounter with the Tulsa police was not the first time he had exhibited strange behavior.

"Something's wrong with Father," a young woman had told the secretary at Saints Peter and Paul Catholic Church in Tulsa. Paul had been counseling the woman and suddenly started to talk gibberish. "He's just not making sense!"

Pastor Kenneth Fulton, associate pastor Father Stieferman, and the secretary immediately went looking for Paul. They found him in the yard staring at the sky.

Father Fulton drove him to Tulsa's Saint Francis Hospital, what would be one of many trips by Paul to local hospitals. My parents were then contacted, and they received a litany of strange stories involving Paul lying prostrate in yards and staring at the sun. A hospital document would later state that my brother had slipped "into a state of catatonic withdrawal."

Paul began to see Dr. Donald Inbody, a Tulsa psychiatrist who had an office at Saint Francis Hospital. Inbody, a longtime parishioner of Saint Mary's in Tulsa, told one priest that Paul's mind was deteriorating, a little more after each catatonic episode. Doctors also believed Paul's prolonged staring at the sun was further damaging his eyes, and they feared he might go blind. Those fears were justified. Paul's eyesight did fail, and although he did not go blind, the lenses of his glasses were like pop-bottle glass.

The initial diagnosis was that Paul was suffering from symptoms caused by either severe stress or, more seriously, a chemical imbalance in the brain. As my parents searched for a clue as to what might have caused the latter, my father learned that Paul might have been slipped LSD once while playing guitar for a youth group. The psychedelic drug became popular in the Sixties, during a time when former Harvard psychologist Timothy Leary was encouraging American students to "turn on, tune in, and drop out," LSD, or acid, is derived from a chemical found in parasitic fungus that grows on rye and other grains, known as ergot. Discovered in 1943 by a Swiss chemist, LSD can cause catatonic states and drug-induced psychosis, with hallucinations and paranoia that mimics schizophrenia.

Unfortunately, at the time my brother fell ill, doctors did not know that LSD's effects were usually only short term and so likely not the reason for Paul's worsening mental condition. My family's belief, however, that Paul had a "chemical imbalance" continued for years and would be recited often as the cause of his health problems.

Conventional wisdom at the time was that a deficiency of serotonin in the brain could cause depression, panic attacks, anxiety disorders, and other forms of mental illness. A later study found that such imbalances could cause higher levels of aggression and psychopathic behavior in a person. Although rare, we now also know that LSD can cause distressing flashbacks of visual hallucinations, a condition called hallucinogen persisting perception disorder, despite no further use of the drug. To this day, however, modern psychiatry and science have yet to definitively prove whether chemical imbalance is a real condition. Some think the claim is a myth/marketing campaign designed to allow pharmaceutical companies to sell large quantities of certain drugs by claiming they can correct such imbalances despite no laboratory test existing for such a condition. The words *schizophrenia* or *paranoid schizophrenia* to describe Paul's condition would not be used until later.

Paul's episodes, meanwhile, became more frequent. After each incident, he would be committed for a short period at Saint Francis and later Hillcrest Hospital, in south Tulsa. On days when he wasn't staring at the sun, Paul could often be found wandering the streets of Tulsa or talking to the voices in his head.

At that time, thorazine, lithium, and other antipsychotic drugs were being used to stabilize patients so they could be released back into the community. The use of prescribed antipsychotic drugs also led to the deinstitutionalization of people with mental illness. The number of people with mental illness in institutions steadily decreased from 560,000 in the mid-1960s to 130,000 by 1980—a fourfold decrease.

Paul was one of many people caught in an endless cycle: Take medication, stop medication, reach crisis, enter jail/crisis center/hospital, stabilize by drugs, release, then reach another crisis. Paul said he stopped taking his medications because the voices told him to quit, but the horrible side effects—restlessness, weight gain, anxiety, and sleep problems—might also have been a factor. The drugs also seemed to trigger other addictive behaviors such as smoking.

Paul began to shy away from crowded rooms. Despite smoking being accepted at the time almost everywhere, he would use it as an excuse to step outside and take a brief walk, especially when he was experiencing anxiety brought on by the drugs. Stopping his medication was not an option. Those same drugs were the only escape from the voices that, although sometimes entertaining, mostly haunted him.

A year after arriving at Saints Peter and Paul, Paul and Stieferman were transferred again in 1971. Stieferman said he was sent to Saint Jude's as a temporary administrator so Father Allen could be treated for alcoholism. Paul became the chaplain at Hillcrest Hospital at Eleventh and Utica that May. Paul was listed as a priest in residence, a designation for priests with duties outside the parish, at the Church of the Madalene, a parish in midtown Tulsa where Father John Sullivan, our old family friend, was pastor.

Except for his receding gray hair and heavier frame, Father Sullivan hadn't changed much since his days at Saint Mary's Church in Guthrie. He still liked to smoke a pipe, and he remained outgoing, well read, and more likely to be seen smiling than not. But most important to Paul, the pastor was supportive of fellow priests who had health issues. And he knew Paul, and I can't help wondering if that had something to do with Paul's new assignment.

Sullivan's powerful post as episcopal vicar in eastern Oklahoma was only one of two in the Oklahoma diocese, and it was seen then as a second in command to the bishop himself. Did this kind, powerful priest step in to give my brother a place to land when maybe others were reluctant? Some priests thought so. One of those who did was Father Patrick J. Gaalaas, who met Paul while preparing for ordination in 1972. He remembers Paul, in a short-sleeved clergy shirt and collar, being on duty at the time.

"Sullivan must have taken Paul under his wing," said Gaalaas. "He knew Paul and liked him." Gaalaas himself would go on to be a vicar general and monsignor.

If all had been well with Paul, he and Sullivan would still have been a fine match. Besides having lived in Guthrie, they had other things in common: Both had a rich Irish heritage and had completed studies at Kendrick Seminary in Saint Louis. Sullivan had also watched Paul grow up, had coached him in basketball, and might well have been involved in recommending that my brother begin studies for the priesthood as a boy. They were both good-natured men who liked to gently tease people and enjoyed a home-cooked meal. And like Paul, Father Sullivan had not only enjoyed his role as a parish priest in a community but also still cherished it. So much so that the coat of arms on Sullivan's vestments commemorated his labors as a priest.

They were brought together during an interesting time for both. Paul was facing personal turmoil, something Gaalaas said my brother never denied and was never resentful of, only "humbly accepting of." Meanwhile, Sullivan—along with Bishop Reed and the Oklahoma Church—was dealing with turmoil of another kind in the wake of Vatican II and other changes happening in the country, such as the civil rights movement. The national press was covering such stories, but at least in Oklahoma, those critical turning points in the Oklahoma Church were going mostly unreported in the Catholic community because its Catholic publications had ceased to exist.

The Oklahoma Courier had become so controversial that the pastoral board, comprised of laypeople and clergy who served at the behest of Bishop Reed, had ordered the newspaper shut down in April 1969. *The Courier* closed even though the bishop himself had said he loved it. The closure came a year after the Tulsa Catholic Center folded its influential newspaper, *At the Center*, which had previously been mailed to area Catholics and nonCatholics alike and considered a pipeline to the National Council of Churches. A Catholic newspaper wouldn't be published in Oklahoma again until 1974, when a much tamer *Sooner Catholic* was launched under the editorship of Father David Monahan. (Monahan died in 2010 after a long decline due to Alzheimer's.) But before all that, *Courier* editor Father John Joyce had already founded another publication, the liberal-leaning *Oklahoma Observer*.

Priests also continued to leave the clergy at alarming rates, with some announcing their intentions openly to their parishioners. Many were notable leaders, including Father Robert Caldwell, head of Catholic Charities in Tulsa, who like so many others left the priesthood to marry. Social justice issues were also coming to the fore. When a wealthy Catholic oilman proposed selling Holy Family Cathedral in downtown Tulsa and building a new cathedral in southeast Tulsa in 1971, Reed quickly withdrew the request in the face of protests by Catholics and priests alike. They opposed the idea of moving out of downtown when needs were mounting in nearby north Tulsa. Father Skeehan went so far as to send a letter protesting the move to every priest in the diocese and to the *National Catholic Reporter*.

Bishop Reed was also pressing ahead with Vatican II reforms, including how mass was celebrated. The liturgical experiments were endless: folk music, drama productions, films, and lectures on "controversial social-action orientation." The changes caused so much turmoil in some parishes that Saint Joseph's, in the college town of Norman, Oklahoma, took a vote to determine whether parishioners liked the new Sunday Mass liturgy at 9:30 a.m. The vote came in 164 to 33 in favor of the new liturgy, but almost a hundred parishioners did not vote.

In yet another unexpected change in the Oklahoma Church, Reed was pushing Rome for Oklahoma City to become an archdiocese so Tulsa could be a diocese of its own. According to the Code of Canon Law, an archdiocese, often called a metropolitan see or the head diocese of an ecclesiastical province, exists to foster cooperation and common pastoral action with a region. Although an archbishop has immediate jurisdiction only over his own diocese, he is charged with several special duties, one of which is to inform the pope in the case of any abuse or neglect in a diocese in his province.

Then on September 8, 1971, the Oklahoma Church was rocked by news concerning its own bishop. After presiding over a meeting of the pastoral board at the Oklahoma City chancery, Bishop Reed had excitedly accepted an invitation to attend a local showing of the movie *Billy Jack* at Quail Twin Theater. During the movie, Monsignor Don J. Kanaly and Father Paul Gallatin noticed the bishop had slumped over in his seat. Assuming that he had simply fallen asleep, they tried to wake him, but Reed was unresponsive. The bishop was rushed to Oklahoma City's Baptist Memorial Hospital, where he received his last rites.

The Oklahoma-reared man who became the fourth bishop in the state and leader of nearly 116,000 Catholics, who was considered among the leaders of Vatican II reforms, who led one of the country's most progressive dioceses, and who became the first American bishop to question the Vietnam War publicly, was soon pronounced dead. Although some Catholic leaders would disagree, Father James D. White wrote in *Tulsa: This Far by Faith*:

> Bishop Reed himself came under vituperative attack from angry Catholics, and the pain that he suffered probably contributed to his early death at sixty-five.

Paul was among some 1,700 mourners on Saturday, September 12, 1971, who attended Bishop Reed's funeral at Tulsa's downtown Holy Family Cathedral, the parish where Reed had previously served for eleven years. Father Sullivan delivered the sermon for his longtime friend, calling the bishop a "man of peace," a civil rights advocate who defended priests arrested with black protesters, and a leader of the ecumenical and reform movement in the country. Sullivan also reminded those gathered that Bishop Reed had been a reconciler who signed a note for an $8,000 loan to start an antiwar movement in 1970. Even though "few people appreciated this man," Sullivan said, "he had a tremendous impact on all who knew him." A second funeral Mass was held the following Monday at the Cathedral of Our Lady of Perpetual Help in Oklahoma City. All Catholic schools in the state were closed that day.

If Pope Paul VI had followed Pope John XXIII's 1958 example in naming Reed, a Tulsa pastor, as bishop, an Oklahoma priest was next in line to become the Oklahoma City–Tulsa Diocese's fifth bishop. If that priest was Father Sullivan, then Paul would have a strong proponent in his now ongoing struggle with mental illness.

Instead, in November 1971, native Californian John Raphael Quinn became the youngest bishop in the country at the age of forty-two when he was named to lead the Oklahoma City–Tulsa Diocese. With no Catholic newspaper left in the state to share the news that day, the *Oklahoma Journal* ran a forty-page special section on Quinn's appointment in which the new bishop declared, "I'm an Oklahoman now." The article also included another bit of news: Quinn would not be opposed to splitting the Oklahoma City–Tulsa Diocese.

If Paul had any hope of returning to central Oklahoma as a priest, a new archdiocese in Oklahoma City and a diocese in Tulsa might effectively end it. However, for at least the moment, he still had his protector in Father Sullivan and the possibility that Sullivan could be named bishop of a new Tulsa Diocese.

* * * * *

My first memory of Bishop Quinn is from a visit he made to Saint Mary's School in Guthrie shortly after his arrival in Oklahoma. I, the brother of a priest, was asked to perform in a skit for the new bishop, as Paul had done as a child. I played the role of a fisherman in a pair of my father's overalls. I remember shaking Bishop Quinn's hand, but mostly I gawked. I was in awe of the handsome young bishop with his warm, dark eyes and black, slicked-back hair parted on the side. Did I see a little of myself in him? Quinn was also the youngest child of his family and had a brother much older than he. And from what I had heard, like my mother, his mother considered him to be "a very good boy."

I didn't know it then, but I was looking at a bishop who would one day speak out against the death penalty and criticize extremists in the antiabortion movement, who would call on Roman Catholics serving in the armed forces to defy any order to detonate a nuclear weapon, and who would create a housing program to help AIDS patients remain in their apartments. That was all yet to come, as was so much more for Quinn, for the American Church, and for my brother, who asked only to be allowed to serve out his calling.

In Tulsa, however, Paul's behavior had become more erratic since Father Sullivan took him in at the Roman Catholic Church of the Madalene, on the corner of East Twenty-Second Street and South Harvard Avenue. Built in 1948, the church had a modern utilitarian design, with a chapel filled with brightly colored stained-glass windows depicting Jesus preaching the Beatitudes from the Sermon on the Mount. The inviting moral code of the Beatitudes was etched in the chapel windows:

> Blessed are the poor in spirit . . . Blessed are those who mourn . . . Blessed are the meek . . . Blessed are those who hunger and thirst for righteous . . . Blessed are the merciful . . . Blessed are the pure in heart . . . Blessed are the peacemakers . . . Blessed are they which are persecuted . . . Blessed are you when people insult you, persecute you, and falsely say all kinds of evil against you because of me . . . Rejoice and be glad because great is your reward in heaven . . .

Father Sullivan embodied the call to be merciful when he took Paul in. The pastor's hospitality, however, was soon tested. Word came home that Paul had punched out a window at Madalene. He later told Mom and Dad that the voices had told him to fight demons at the church, and he punched out the window because he saw demons in it.

The voices in his head were growing stronger. Before Mass on one Sunday, Paul blocked the entrance as parishioners tried to file into church.

"Don't come in," Paul told them as they approached. "There are demons inside, so we're not having Mass today. Go on home."

Some parishioners were apparently so stunned by Paul's proclamation that they turned around and left without even questioning him. Others, however, reported Paul's behavior to the pastor, and Paul was soon back in the hospital for treatment. Still, Sullivan never wavered as Paul's protector, and he did become a bishop.

* * * * *

In July 1972, Father Sullivan was appointed to head the Grand Island [Nebraska], Diocese, and no one was more shocked by Pope Paul VI's announcement than Sullivan.

"Never have I been so aware of my dependence upon God," the bishop-elect said. "In all candor, I am grieved at leaving Oklahoma and all of my friends I have been associated with, but I look forward to my new responsibilities with a spirit of faith, obedience, and hope."

The news about Sullivan's elevation and new assignment must have devastated Paul—and my parents as well, although Paul did continue on at Madalene. When treatment kept the voices at bay, Paul could perform his priestly duties at the parish and elsewhere, including ecumenical gatherings and those involving family. In 1972, Paul was the chief presider of a backyard wedding for our brother, John, and Jan Larkin. John and Jan had met while attending Oklahoma State University. They had had to receive special permission for the interdenominational wedding, which would include Paul, a Tulsa Catholic priest, and a Baptist minister representing Jan's family. The couple had also gone through the required Catholic premarital counseling from the priest at Saint Mary's in Guthrie. As part of that process, each had completed a long form, which among other questions asked, "Have you ever committed a crime, been diagnosed with a mental illness, or are a nonCatholic?"

"Are all those considered equal?" Jan asked the priest.

She later learned that the priest had reported back to Dad that she was "difficult," an observation my father found hilarious.

Approved to preside over the ceremony, Paul agreed to add his own words and prayers to the vows Jan and John had written. The wedding was set for July 14, which was my fourteenth birthday. John and Jan asked me to be an usher. I made my appearance in a three-button, pale blue suit that, not unlike Paul's priestly vestments, hung loosely on my skinny frame. My straight sandy-blond hair was combed over my fore-head, and photographs from the wedding reveal that I had acquired the awkward smirk of Paul in his teens. As for Paul, having received per-mission to officiate, he was jovial and entertaining through the wedding and the festivities that followed. At one point, when it came time to cue the classical guitarist, Paul did so with the line, "Love does not come to an end," a dramatic bow, and a flourish of the hand.

Photographs, however, record the effects of his mental illness. His hairline had receded, and he had gained weight, perhaps another side effect of his medication. In one photograph, he sits holding a wedding program, but instead of reading, he is staring off into the distance.

Three weeks later, on August 5, he presided over the wedding of our sister Susan to Mike Williams. They, too, had met while at Oklahoma State. (Paul and I were the only ones in our immediate family not to attend OSU.) The temperature that day reached 97 degrees Fahren-heit, and Saint Mary's seemed just as hot inside, but Paul flawlessly per-formed the wedding in the church of his childhood. Once again, family members did not detect in him any signs of mental illness, even though we were now aware of his struggles with it.

A month later, on Tuesday, September 21, 1972, Paul was among 150 Oklahoma priests, a hundred out-of-state priests, nuns from fifteen states, and two thousand members of the laity, including my parents, who crowded into the Tulsa Civic Assembly Center for Father Sullivan's ordination as bishop. The ordination was the first to be held outside an Oklahoma cathedral. Sullivan called it "a magnificent expression, not only of our own unity in faith and friendship, but of the unity of the universal Church."

Two days later, my parents and Paul attended Sullivan's installation in Grand Island, Nebraska, at Saint Mary's Cathedral. Sullivan's priestly journey, which had started at Saint Mary's in Guthrie, Oklahoma, had come full circle. The next day, Cardinal John Cody of Chicago presided over the installation of Sullivan, a man who had spent most of his life in Oklahoma but was destined never to return.

All the pomp and circumstance of the ceremony must have been bittersweet for my parents. I know they were happy that their friend and his gifts were being recognized by the larger Church, but their worry about what that would mean for their son must have been acute.

The announcement that the Oklahoma City–Tulsa Diocese would split came only three months after Sullivan left the state, just before Christmas in 1972. The Archdiocese of Oklahoma City would consist of forty-six counties in western and central Oklahoma and include seventy-one parishes, eighteen in Oklahoma City.

The Tulsa Diocese would include Tulsa and thirty-one counties in eastern Oklahoma. Priests in both dioceses had to make quick choices, Gaalaas said: Go freely to either diocese during the first two weeks or exchange with another priest of equal rank in the following two weeks. A priest struggling with mental illness probably didn't have a choice. Paul would remain in Tulsa for the remainder of his priesthood.

After the split, early in 1973, Bishop Quinn was named archbishop, and another relatively young priest, another outsider, was named bishop of Tulsa: Bernard Ganter, a forty-four-year-old who hailed from the Galveston-Houston Diocese and a Texas A&M graduate. At about the same time, Monsignor Cecil Finn was named pastor of Madalene. With balding blond hair, bushy sideburns, and strong facial features, the new pastor was known for his "astonishing vitality and athleticism" (he played multiple sports, including racquetball, golf, and tennis) and for setting a "lively pace" for his associate pastors. His vigor stood in stark contrast to Paul, who was neither athletic nor particularly energetic as a result of his battle with his mental demons, a fight that both dioceses were now aware was ongoing.

The change in pastors.

The change in bishops.

The changes in his health.

And the departure of John J. Sullivan from Tulsa ended the first of three life-changing cycles for Paul, each thirteen to fifteen years apart. The first cycle started with a request made to the Catholic Church, one that remains mysterious to Paul's family to this day.

Chapter 9

Departure from the Brotherhood

The Catholic Church's crisis of priests seeking to no longer be a priest was beginning to threaten its core. In 1975, Paul would become one of them. Only in his case, a mystery surrounds his departure. Was it his decision to leave the priesthood, or was his exodus forced on him by the Church he loved?

That would seem to be the ultimate contradiction: once a priest, always a priest—until you're not. In practice, the finality of laicization for a priest is absolute and binding, so much so that a former priest is asked by the Church not to live in or frequent places where his former status as a priest is known. He is told not to serve in most capacities with the Catholic Church, such as on parish staff or anything associated with the Church unless he receives permission from the bishop. He is defined as having been "defrocked," or removed from his priestly powers.

In many ways, he becomes an outcast, reversing sacred vows that took him more than a decade of school and training to achieve and that historically were deemed irreversible by the Church itself.

What leaving the priesthood does not necessarily mean is that a priest turns his back on God or even Catholicism, although it might be seen as though he is turning his back on Rome and the Church hierarchy that he previously pledged to serve and obey. In a case such as Paul's, however, it would seem the Catholic Church was turning its back on its own, and the most vulnerable of its own at that.

And then, as a practical matter, could a Catholic Church that was losing priests each and every day afford to cast one out because of his illness, especially at a time when other priests were being actively protected from allegations of sexual abuse against children?

What was true is that after six years in the priesthood, Paul's mental illness was getting worse. That meant more hospitalizations. More strange public incidents. More scrutiny from a Church that frowned upon what they considered unacceptable: the scandal of his behavior. For the last two years of his priesthood, the newly formed archdiocese simply listed Paul in the annual directory as being on "sick leave." Those in the know recognized those words for what they were: a euphemism for a host of conditions, such as an alcoholic priest, a priest suffering from nervous exhaustion, a priest caught in a relationship with a woman, a priest accused of child sex abuse, a disobedient priest.

Nearly 3,100 men left the priesthood in the United States from the time Paul became a priest in 1968 until the time he was facing laicization himself in 1975. In 1967, the United States had 59,892 priests for its 2.3 million Catholics. When Paul became a priest, the number had declined only slightly to 59,803. However, by 1974, 56,712 remained. The priesthood would eventually rebound to 58,485 by 1978, but statistics still show a decline of more than 1,400 from 1967 to 1978. Those statistics also do not consider the possibility that all U.S. dioceses were not properly reporting the number of their departing priests.

The disturbing trend brought a myriad of reactions. In Oklahoma, established priests wrote open letters to young men encouraging them to enter the priesthood. Surveys explored why priests were leaving. At least one archbishop talked openly with his priests about the usually secretive process of laicization and the causes. Archbishop Thomas J. McDonough was two years in as archbishop in Louisville, Kentucky, when he took the extraordinary step in early 1969 of broaching the subject with his priests. Considered a staunch Vatican II advocate, McDonough called laicization a new Church process that "will undergo many modifications until the best process can be worked out."

Unlike more traditional Catholics and clergy, McDonough did not see a priest's decision to leave the priesthood as a threat to the Church or Catholicism but as more of a personal matter. People change. What they want out of their one life changes. What a young man inspires to might not be what he wants in middle age. That the pre–Vatican II Church also put boys on the path to priesthood before some had gone through puberty raises the question as to whether the latter were capable of informed consent. That path brought prestige to themselves and their family, a difficult path to exit for any young man. In an NC News Service interview, McDonough observed:

> The laicization of a priest begins in a man's own inner self, in an attempt to face honesty in his beliefs, his fears, his own honesty, and his God. This comes, usually, after a period of tension, turmoil, prayer, and discussion.

McDonough saw laicization itself as a process that should unfold in a logical and reasonable way:

> At the first meeting the priest should either request a leave of absence or for the archbishop to present a petition to Rome requesting he be removed from his priestly duties. The archbishop should offer financial aid to the priest so he can seek psychiatric treatment if he wants, although most priests reject this because they don't feel they need treatment. After approval is requested from Rome, the priest should be given a leave of absence for several months to a year and be "free to call upon the diocese for any reasonable economic aid or moral support."

The step after the formal leave of absence, McDonough said:

> . . . is a serious one, and the priest considering it should spend some time adjusting to his new social, economic, and ecclesial roles. [However, if the decision is made to seek laicization,] a review of the priest's reasons for asking for a dispensation, and a letter from the archbishop regarding the priest are then sent to Rome.

McDonough realized that the act of leaving the priesthood was perilous. As Father Stieferman had observed earlier, some men left the priesthood thinking that would solve all their problems; that was not always the case. The fate of one priest in his archdiocese dogged McDonough even after the man's death in 1998 as a case of laicization that should have been sought earlier by both him and the Church. Father Louis E. Miller was convicted in 2003 of molesting twenty-one children over decades. In a deposition, Miller testified that in the early 1990s, his therapist had told police that he was a sexual offender, but police never followed up. Five days before his sentencing, Miller testified that three Louisville archbishops, including McDonough, knew about the molestations but kept him in the priesthood. Miller was sentenced to twenty years in prison.

A baffling issue also worth considering was what mental gymnastics had to be exercised to rationalize keeping pedophiles, such as Miller, in the priesthood instead of seeking their laicization earlier. Financial reasons might have been driving the delays. According to a 2004 research study by the John Jay College of Criminal Justice for the U.S. Conference of Catholic Bishops, 4,392 Catholic priests and deacons in active ministry between 1950 and 2002 have been plausibly accused of sexually abusing underage children. Since 2004, nineteen Catholic dioceses and religious orders in the United States have filed for bankruptcy because of the clergy sexual abuse crisis, according to the *National Catholic Reporter*.

The impetus to seek laicization for most priests had nothing to do with abuse or mental illness or being too young when they started on their path to the priesthood. They simply wanted to marry. A survey of 231 former U.S. priests published in the Gallagher Presidents' Report said the average age of priests who were leaving the priesthood was thirty-eight, and they had been in the priesthood for eleven years. Of those, 73 percent named celibacy as the major reason for their departure.

Noted author and researcher Father Joseph Fichte, who spent most of his career at Loyola University in New Orleans and sought to desegregate Catholic schools in the south, advocated for priests marrying. His polls of his fellow priests, *The New York Times* reported in his obituary in 1994, revealed that most priests were in favor of allowing marriage, even those who chose to remain celibate themselves.

Yet Fichte saw problems with priestly formation, the act of training a priest to be a priest. While serving as executive secretary of the American Bishops' Committee on Priestly Formation, he maintained that the Church was plagued by the "functionary priest . . . who goes through the motions." He believed that many priests wanted to do more. His surveys showed 87 percent of younger priests at the time wanted to continue their education and become more professional. More than half of them thought they were working below capacity. "We have more functionaries, more job holders, than professionals among the Catholic clergy today," Fichte told a gathering of New England's bishops and religious leaders at the time, "and that is the Church's central problem—not birth control, or abortion, or celibacy, or Catholic schools."

Those not challenged by their work are prone to "boredom and frustration." Fichte blamed Church leaders for the problems, claiming he didn't believe a shortage of priests existed. "Only bad management," he said. "Management knows that it is much easier to handle job holders than to manage professionals—and this point must be kept in mind."

The Official Catholic Directory annually tracks the total number of priests, active priests, resident priests not considered active but who live in a rectory or reside within a parish, and retired, sick, or absent priests. Paul would eventually be classified in every category except retired or absent. When he became a priest in 1968, the Oklahoma City–Tulsa Diocese had 281 priests, 181 active priests, seventy in-residence priests, seventeen active priests living outside the diocese, and thirteen retired, sick, or absent ones. The Catholic population in Oklahoma at the time was 112,127.

By Paul's second year in the priesthood, the total number of priests had risen to 290. By 1972, the last year that statistics were kept for the diocese, when 116,608 resident Oklahomans were Catholics, the total had dropped in three years by twenty-six priests. During the first year of the Oklahoma City Archdiocese and Tulsa Diocese, thirty-seven men left the priesthood. In the second year, 1974, eleven more left, before the number of Oklahoma clergy stabilized in 1975 at 242 priests. The number of Oklahoma Catholics also dropped to 108,668 in 1974 and then to 106,266 in 1975. The state's Catholic population rebounded in 1978 to 113,593, but the number of priests did not, falling to 239. In 1980, the Oklahoma City and Tulsa dioceses had only 236 priests for 117,563 Catholics.

The crisis also prompted one priest to submit an open letter in *The Oklahoma Courier* to potential future priests. Father Bernard J. Havlik, who was in Tonkawa at the time, had been a priest for twenty-five years, and he urged future and fellow priests to "keep our commitment as priests ever before our minds." He wrote:

> The temptations to leave the priesthood for any other type of job or to get married never really entered my mind, though perhaps on fleeting occasion such thoughts did enter therein. It was without doubt the grace of God and the prayers of the members of my family and friends which kept me from entertaining such thoughts. . . .
>
> What I really wanted to write to you courageous young men (no one can deny that it takes a lot more courage nowadays to want to become a priest than it did twenty-five years ago) is to urge each of you to cultivate a manly attachment to prayer, prayer that is both official and private. Such an attachment to prayer in my

estimation help(s) keep the goals of the priesthood and above all of its obligations always before our minds."

Havlik's advice was good, but it failed to stem the exodus of priests. Yet another Oklahoma priest's departure came in May 1973. Father Dean Schlecht, associate pastor of Saint John's University Parish in Stillwater, told his parishioners that he would be leaving the priesthood to marry an Oklahoma State University doctoral student. The twist to his announcement: He would be visiting a canon lawyer in Oklahoma City to draft a letter asking the Catholic Church in Rome if he could marry. "Obviously, I think the Church should allow married clergy," Schlecht said at the time. "Rome and the hierarchy are making a severe mistake in their rejection of optional celibacy."

Schlecht, who had spent four years at Saint John's, voluntarily resigned from the Church and his parish post but still wanted to seek permission to marry. He and Carol Davenport wanted to marry in his former parish. At the time, Schlecht thought it would take nine months to receive a reply from Rome.

In many ways, Schlecht's priesthood mirrored Paul's except that he had been ordained a year earlier, in 1967, and entered at thirteen years of age. As Paul had, Schlecht first attended a minor seminary in Bethany before then leaving for high school and further studies in San Antonio. The early priestly education had left him bitter about the process.

"The concept of [a] minor seminary is bizarre," Schlecht said many years later. "It's inappropriate to take a child away from his family and put him into a boarding school. It does enormous harm and is an enormous waste of money. Only one in twenty go on to become priests."

The Associated Press news service covered Schlecht's announcement, but my brother's decision to leave the priesthood drew no such press, although Paul was going through the same process for different reasons. From 1973 through 1974, Paul remained listed as on sick leave in diocesan directories. A careful observer would have noticed that his last known address as a priest was the same post office box as the diocese's chancery office.

Paul's leave request was not a protest of Catholic theology and did not stem from a desire to marry. Mental illness caused Paul's request. Without his old family friend, now-Bishop Sullivan in Nebraska, Paul had no one in the Church to turn to for support. A few other priests tried to help him, but none had enough power to stop the inevitable. As Schlecht would say later, the Church is "invested in power and control. It's there to protect the institution rather than facilitate grace." Schlecht remembered little about Paul but knew he had had mental health struggles. "He was a quiet and gentle person," said Schlecht, who went on to run a psychiatric crisis respite facility in Oregon.

As the end of Paul's time in the priesthood drew near, Dad made a short, matter-of-fact announcement to Mom and me: "Paul apparently sent a letter to Rome asking to be laicized. He may be moving home soon." My parents seemed resigned to Paul's fate, convinced that his undoing stemmed from a chemical imbalance and his frequent erratic behavior. As the years passed, however, questions arose as to whether the request had been Paul's choice or whether the new leadership in the Tulsa Diocese had made the choice for him.

A priest's file is highly confidential even after death, when those records are moved to a diocese's secret archives where only a bishop can authorize their release. They are not readily available to family. Years later, the Tulsa Diocese initially released an outline of the records and letters contained in Paul's file and then twelve of the forty-one documents considered "public." They show a trail starting when Paul entered the seminary in 1963. But the most interesting parts begin in 1973. Although the diocesan directory listed him as being on sick leave, one document showed he was named associate pastor of Christ the King Parish effective March 30, 1973. The records also seemed to indicate that Paul had a different ministry while on sick leave and that the bishop thought he was well when making the appointment.

"This is to be a full-time assignment to the parish, and hence I ask that you discontinue the work you had been doing in the various nursing homes. Each parish can take care of its own," Bishop Bernard Ganter wrote in a March 26 letter sent to an address in a quiet Tulsa neighborhood. "I am grateful to God that He has restored your health so that you will be able to accept this assignment and do his work. You can do so much for the Lord for you have the talent and zeal. I would also ask that you do not push yourself too much. It is important that we learn to pace ourselves."

Gaalaas said he thought Ganter had been named bishop because of his administrative experience after previously being a chancellor/vicar general. He remembers the bishop as a quiet, thoughtful man who was known for fasting—and for his notes. Just before his death in 1993, Ganter, as bishop of Beaumont, Texas, sent Gaalaas a nice note congratulating him for becoming the Tulsa diocese chancellor.

Paul remained at Christ the King for only six months until he was named associate pastor at Holy Family Cathedral. That same month, the diocese addressed "medical bills" and opened an account in Paul's name at Tulsa Federal Savings in Tulsa. Father Elkin Gonzalez, vicar general for the Tulsa Diocese in 2017 when the outline was released, said Paul might have been moved again that year to accommodate his mental illness in the hopes of finding a more understanding pastor at a different parish.

To this day, the family has no copy or record of any letter from Paul to Rome or the diocese requesting laicization. The outline does show that Paul signed a letter of request for a leave of absence on May 6, 1974, but does not indicate whose idea that was, Paul's or someone else's. Two days later, Bishop Ganter accepted the letter. The released documents show the bishop tried to reach Paul at a Tulsa apartment complex in early October to "have the opportunity to visit with you and see how things are going. . . . You have often been in my thoughts and prayers." The outline then shows the bishop received a memo dated October 15 regarding Paul's location.

In December, a McAlester woman who described herself as Paul's "friend" asked for his address because she wanted to "let him know we will be thinking of him during the coming holidays." The diocese sent her an address in northwest Tulsa, a different address than the October one in southwest Tulsa.

Only a few people knew Paul had moved home to Guthrie.

My brother's journey out of the priesthood was nearing an end by June 9, 1975, when Diocesan Chancellor Father Joseph Propps requested information about Paul from psychiatrist Dr. Inbody and Father Thomas Biller. Why Biller's name was included in the correspondence is not clear, although he had been a former associate pastor with Paul at Madalene.

About that same time, Paul also wrote a note authorizing Father Propps's request for information from Dr. Inbody and Father Biller. By the next month, on July 15, insurance claims for Paul's past hospitalizations had been submitted to the diocese. A priest under review by his diocese is supposed to have access to a canon lawyer, but documents do not indicate whether Paul was ever granted this. Father Gonzalez, however, said the process seemed amiable in his review of the documents.

The "official petition for laicization" on Paul's behalf went off to Rome. On July 22, 1975, a response came back from the Congregation for the Doctrine of Faith, the official body for defending Catholic doctrine and enforcing canon law, also known as the Holy Office. At the time, the Holy Office was also considering whether sterilizations should be allowed in Catholic hospitals. A year later, Rome would rule that women shouldn't be admitted to the priesthood because of the historic tradition of the Catholic Church, even though "women have played a decisive role and accomplished tasks of outstanding value."

The Congregation for the Doctrine of Faith is known to handle "processes that are more 'penal' in nature," according to a 2010 story in *The Catholic Sun*. The congregation deals with priests accused of the sexual abuse of minors or a cleric judged unfit for public ministry because of some other circumstance or act. In Paul's case, the congregation might have been trying to determine whether Paul had a recognized impediment or irregularity covered by canon law.

Today, under the 1983 Code of Canon Law, irregularities that can prevent a person from becoming or serving as a priest include having committed heresy, mutilated himself, attempted marriage, or participated in a murder or an abortion. Mental illness tops the list as a condition that prevents the fulfillment of the priestly duties.

But in 1974 the congregation was governed by the 1917 Code of Canon Law, so the Holy Office would have been reviewing a list of more dramatic possibilities to determine whether Paul's impediment meant he was unfit for the priesthood: "Those who are or were epileptics, insane, or possessed by the devil impaired in body."

Tellingly, the 1917 Code of Law also noted, "But if after reception of orders they fall into these and it is certainly proved that they are freed, the Ordinary can permit his subjects to exercise once again the orders already received."

That begs the question: If Paul had taken his medication regularly, could he have continued as a priest? Or maybe equally important, did the Oklahoma Church even explore that option? There are many and varied ways for a priest who falls ill to serve—visiting the sick or elderly or engaging in devotional prayer among them.

The congregation's prefect is one of the most powerful leadership positions in the Catholic Church; in 1975, the nearly seventy-year-old Croatian Cardinal Franjo Seper had held the position for seven years. He would remain in the position until November 1981 and then die a month later. His successor, Cardinal Joseph Ratzinger, a good friend of Pope John Paul II, would one day become Pope Benedict XVI and then in 2013, the first pontiff in six centuries to abdicate the papacy.

As noted earlier, canon law states that a priest who validly receives "sacred ordination" remains a priest for life. However, a priest can lose his clerical state, which means he can no longer act as a priest, celebrate Mass, be called Reverend or Father, or be supported by the Church. He can still administer the Last Rites, including confession, to a dying person—1917 canon law referred to it as "The Reduction of Clerics to the Lay State," but that wording later was changed so as not to infer that laity was an inferior state.

Because of Vatican II, in Paul's day, canon law was constantly under debate and evolving. By 1971, the "responsible agent" for submitting a petition was changed to the priest's bishop. According to the *Catholic Encyclopedia*, in 1972, the congregation then sent a letter that stated the following:

Laicization should never be the first, but only the last resort in salvaging a disintegrated priestly commitment; and ordinaries are encouraged to use every means to help prevent a priest from seeking a dispensation on impulse, in a state of depression, or without truly mature and solid motivation. Current canon law dictates an irregularity as being a "person who labors under some form of amentia or other psychic illness due to which, after experts have been consulted, he is judged unqualified to fulfill the ministry properly."

Amentia is defined as a "severe mental handicap," or what was formerly known as "mental retardation."

In the 1970s, Pope Paul VI was supposed to have the final say. More likely, the congregation merely verified what Bishop Ganter stated or requested in the petition for laicization. Monsignor Dennis Dorney, a friend of Paul's and former Tulsa Diocese vicar general, said the process in 1974 would have called for Paul to submit a letter to the bishop, and then Ganter would have forwarded the letter to the Vatican. But no such letter exists in the diocese's files or my brother's personal papers. In the "straightforward and simple" process described by Schlecht, Paul did meet before his leave of absence with Bishop Ganter.

Paul described his one-on-one meeting with the bishop to the same Father Denis Hanrahan who became his friend and confidant years later. As Hanrahan recalled:

> Paul asked, What about retirement?
> You will not receive it, the bishop replied.
> What about insurance?
> We will take care of you, Ganter replied.

"What one bishop said, another changed," Hanrahan said. "He was encouraged by the Diocese of Tulsa to seek laicization. My understanding from Paul is that they encouraged him to seek laicization."

Monsignor Dorney added, "He was laicized because it was obviously endorsed by the bishop. He was unable to function in a normal capacity as a priest. You can be laicized for mental and emotional health reasons." Dorney said that in 1974, the Church didn't have the capacity to deal with someone with severe mental illness. "It still doesn't."

In trying to explain what Paul had done to run afoul of his superiors, Dorney mentioned Paul's catatonic episodes, but Dorney also talked about Paul's habitual giving, which irritated his fellow priests. According to the monsignor, at least one priest "got onto to him for giving away all of his money. . . . Paul would give his money to anyone who knocked on the door and asked." That behavior continued after Paul moved out of the rectory. Tulsa police would call to say that Paul was taking food out of trash cans at a restaurant or was being evicted from an apartment because he couldn't pay the rent. The reason: He had no money left after having given away what little he had to others.

No matter how, Paul's tenure as a member of the clergy was over after a little more than six years, officially seven years, after his ordination. On October 24, 1975, the Holy Office sent a decree of laicization for Paul to a small home in southwest Tulsa. Written entirely in Latin, the decree stated that he had "been reduced to the lay state." The document removed him from most priestly duties and supposedly barred him from receiving any assistance from the diocese or the Church. "When you've been laicized by Rome, you're not entitled to any compensation from the diocese," Dorney said. "They might [have] provide[d] assistance if he were having trouble getting medicine. I don't remember that he did."

For the first time since he was a teenager, Paul was separated from the Church that he had vowed to serve and that he thought had pledged itself to him. There was no elaborate ceremony as there had been when he was ordained, and not any formality either, nothing to mark the fact that a thirty-two-year-old man had lost the foundation of his life.

Schlecht also would leave the priesthood but at age thirty-one. He never did receive a response to his letter asking the Vatican hierarchy if he could marry. "There was an awful lot of people leaving at the time. Maybe they were overwhelmed with the requests and just stuffed mine in a drawer." Schlecht would later become a psychotherapist, and unlike many of his peers, he also left the Catholic Church, an institution he calls a "major disappointment . . . driving itself downhill. The clergy sexual abuse scandal is an example." The former priest went on to write the book *Embracing the Self* about where he landed after abandoning Catholicism. "My spirituality evolved," Schlecht said, ". . . and has nothing to do with dogma or group affiliation."

In the case of my brother, the Catholic Church left him. Paul would never fully leave the Church nor fully give up his role as a priest to others. How he was treated by the Church, however, still elicits sympathy from several priests from his time and has left others embittered. Before his passing in 2016, Father Stieferman talked at length about many issues from that turbulent time in the Oklahoma Church until he was asked, *Why didn't the Church take care of Paul?*

His calm manner turned angry. He shared that another priest, a manic depressive, had received support. "I really disagreed with that decision [about Paul]. They took care of other priests. They should have taken care of him," Stieferman said. "I don't think they should have kicked him out. He wasn't in any shape to write a letter [to Rome] anyway. That was cruel."

Hanrahan agreed, "It was a wrong decision. That relieved them of all responsibility—to [cover Paul's] insurance and salary every month."

The Church's treatment of a gentle, ill priest such as Paul would have bothered anyone who follows Matthew 25:40:

> Whatever you did for one of these least brothers of mine, you did for me.

What haunted me was how Paul's expulsion from the priesthood stood in stark contrast to so many other cases. About the same time that Paul was going through laicization in 1974, Father Richard Frank Dolan, a recovering alcoholic, was arrested and charged with engaging in an act of lewdness with an Oklahoma City vice squad officer. The police had established a sting operation focusing on gay prostitution in an area near downtown. The target: the prostitutes' customers. Forty-one-year-old Dolan was the first arrest. Dolan went on to operate several controversial bingo halls in Oklahoma City in the late 1970s. Yet despite his brushes with the law, Dolan always remained popular with fellow priests.

"He was a very charming fellow," Father Monahan, the respected Oklahoma City Archdiocese spokesman and *Sooner Catholic* editor, said after Dolan's 1988 murder, which remains unsolved. "I hope people will remember him for all the good he did."

And Dolan did do good. The year Paul was ordained in 1968, Dolan established The Main Artery for alcoholics. The one-armed priest had been appointed the year before as the diocesan delegate for rehabilitation of alcoholics and was allowed to use a Catholic building in Tulsa to begin The Main Artery.

Yet the tolerance shown by the Oklahoma City Archdiocese for a priest suffering from alcoholism and problems with the law apparently did not extend to a young Tulsa priest suffering from mental illness. Stories circulated among Oklahoma priests as to the whereabouts of my brother after he left the priesthood and what he ended up doing after hanging up his collar. Some had him working at a casket company. Others thought he was homeless and living out of restaurant trash cans.

In truth, Paul simply returned home to Guthrie, but this time, not as a seminarian or the perfect priest.

Chapter 10

The Shadow

Paul returned home in 1974, but the mood stood in stark contrast from his triumphant visits as a young priest. Gone were the exuberant smile and booming voice that rivaled our father's. In their stead was a tall man, still in his early thirties but so hunched over he could have been mistaken for a man in his eighties. In the past on his visits, Paul had often brought gifts of candy or trinkets, often religious in nature, which I looked forward to, as did our mother.

This time, I dreaded his arrival.

My parents had told me enough that I knew Paul was no longer a priest and that he had suffered another breakdown. The night before my parents brought him home, and for many nights to this day, I dreamed that our doors were not properly shut and locked and that we were vulnerable to intruders. In the dream, I am in a panic as I try to close the doors only to have them creak open again and again. Nothing I do keeps them closed and us safe. And then I wake up.

Paul's return home was reminiscent of that nightmare, only this time, my parents were the ones who had unlocked the door and allowed the stranger to enter our home. The person I had emulated all my life was suddenly not only no longer the person I wanted to become but also someone I feared. My parents and I would need time to adjust, but Mom and Dad began to realize what they faced, as every parent of a child with paranoid schizophrenia of any age does: a life sentence as a caregiver of an adult child.

Paul reentered my life during what had been until then my carefree teenage years. After sharing a bedroom with older brothers for what felt like forever, I finally had my own room. And one of the benefits of being the last child at home meant that I had inherited the bigger, back-corner bedroom in our four-bedroom house. Paul was assigned to the middle bedroom in the hallway next to mine.

Until then, I had not noticed much of a difference in my big brother, even after the onset of his bouts with mental illness. Now, however, I noticed Paul seemed off, rarely making eye contact, always looking into the distance, and frowning constantly. Soon, Dad seemed irritated that Paul was home, and Mom took to wearing a concerned expression that made her look older than her years. I couldn't help wondering if Paul saw what I saw, and if so, did his parents' new attitude toward him hurt or worry him? It certainly worried me.

As the days pushed forward, a disturbing trend began. Paul would get up in the middle of the night and wander around the house. I would hear him stomp out the front or back door to smoke a cigarette, walk the roadways, or pace the front yard. When asked about this late-night activity, he shrugged it off as the side effects of his medication, although I knew Dad blamed it on Paul *not* taking his medication as he should.

Sometimes Paul remained inside, pacing from the utility room at one end of the house to the other, which happened to be the bathroom next to my bedroom. I tried to sleep through his restlessness but often failed. Many a night, I was still awake at midnight, with the sound of Paul's incessant pacing the only noise in the house. His steps would fade, but then grow louder and louder until finally a shadow the size of a grizzly bear would stop in front of my open bedroom door. Paul would linger there, staring inside. He never said a word at such times, nor did he ever enter my bedroom. His presence recalled his pranks during my childhood, when Paul would appear at my bedroom window and making haunting sounds in a deep voice like Vincent Price. I found his silence and this new shadow much more menacing.

In other ways, I was experiencing a weird sense of role reversal with my older brother. Summer was on us and had brought weeds to pull, vegetables to pick, and lawns to be mowed, although when I could, I slept in late. Early one morning, however, I was awakened by my father shouting: "Joe, get up! I need you to clean out the greenhouse today."

Dad had been muttering that he needed to retire and end the drudgery of the daily forty-plus-minute carpool drive to Midwest City and the Air Logistics Center when suddenly he barked the most surprising of orders on his way out: "Find Paul! You can tell him what to do."

A newfound sense of power washed over me—I had the authority to tell my oldest brother what to do. I sprang out of bed, dressed quickly, and began to search for my newly assigned subordinate.

"Paul! Paul!" I screamed as I ran out the front door.

I found my oldest brother smoking a cigarette near the mimosa tree in our front yard, the smoke drifting away on a gusty wind. I told him that Dad said we had to clean up the greenhouse and, almost with glee, added that he had put me in charge. That news appeared to anger Paul at first, but he didn't say a word. Instead, he walked over to the driveway, threw the cigarette down, and purposefully grounded the butt into the concrete.

Disapproval could trigger Paul's anxiety, and our mother did not approve of his smoking, so usually he would walk away, out of sight of the house, to smoke. When he was *off*, as we called it, Paul became more brazen, sometimes smoking in front of the living room's big picture window so our mother could see him. As Paul finished grinding that cigarette into the drive, I looked up to see my mother standing in the picture window, watching him, the most inscrutable look on her face. She did not acknowledge that she saw me. Paul lumbered toward the greenhouse, and I followed. Weeds and vegetation had overgrown the greenhouse, and shards of clay pots and trash covered the floor. Dust from months of winter neglect covered everything.

Exercising my newfound authority, I told Paul to sweep the green-house. Paul did as he was told, while I mostly played supervisor. Paul didn't speak for the next few hours, as he swept and then began to pick up trash. He occasionally lifted his head to stare at me, and then he would nod his head and smile broadly, as if the voices were talking to him. I knew something was wrong, but my self-satisfaction in my new role as boss blinded me as to what it might be. I just kept pushing Paul to work faster, while I did little to help.

At lunchtime, we devoured the sandwiches Mom had made for us so we could finish up and maybe avoid the late-afternoon summer heat. But by midafternoon, we were still at it. The sun was now bearing down hard on the greenhouse, making the inside ten degrees hotter than out-side. I told Paul it was time for a water break and headed to the house, where I immediately began to prepare a glass of ice water, for me. I heard Mom putting clothes into the washer in the utility room but not my brother come in from outside.

And then I heard my mother scream, "Paul!"

With glass in hand, I turned to find Paul standing about six feet behind me. His eyes were wild, and once again he was smiling broadly. His right hand was raised and held a kitchen knife—to this day I don't know how he got it without my hearing him.

I dropped my glass and it shattered on the floor. Paul did not flinch, and what happened next seemed in slow motion. He stared at me as if he were waiting on the order for what to do next, and when I didn't give him one, he began to frown. I glanced at the knife he still held and then into his blank eyes. Part of me thought maybe he was playing around, trying to scare me, so I smirked and asked if he needed a drink of water. Nothing. I asked if he needed something. Still, nothing. I asked if he wanted me to put the knife away. Again, nothing. He just continued to stare into my eyes. And then suddenly, he moved toward me.

"Paul, what are you doing?" Mother screamed again.

Her words pierced the room, and, for the first time, I realized that the knife was intended for me. I fell back against the counter, with Paul still halfway across the room near the back door.

My mother's scream, however, had broken whatever had held my brother in its sway. Paul shook his head, as if coming out of a deep sleep. His eyes changed from blank to recognition. He glanced at me and then turned and looked at Mom. Paul must have read the terror in her eyes, although she spoke not a word. He put the knife on the counter and walked out the door.

My mother quickly retrieved the knife and returned it to its proper place, and then went back to loading the wet clothes into the hamper.

Not another word was said.

The kitchen floor remained covered in broken glass.

Almost half a century later, as with Paul's dream about heaven and hell, I still remember every detail of that afternoon, but I have never believed Paul intended to hurt me. The knife was simply visual intimidation to end what he perceived as a threat from an authority figure, this time a brother nearly sixteen years younger than he was, a mere boy.

If intimidation had indeed been his plan, it worked. My workday was over, even though the unfinished greenhouse chores remained. Paul's response to our encounter was to return to the greenhouse and continue to work but without someone half his age telling him what to do. My response was to retreat to my room, where I sank into a deep sleep. No one said anything to me for several days about what had happened in our kitchen. Dad was the one who finally broached the subject with me, acknowledging how upset my mother was. He admitted that he didn't understand what Paul had been up to. I said Paul was probably angry with me for ordering him about in the greenhouse.

Dad made it clear what had happened was not my fault but said I needed to be careful when Paul wasn't in his right mind. I don't know why, but in the end, the incident didn't affect me any more than Paul's mischievous attempts to scare me had when I was younger.

Paul's late-night visits to my bedroom door continued through the summer. They weren't life-threatening, but they did make an impression. When soon thereafter I started to close my bedroom door at night, I saw it as a sign that I was leaving childhood fears behind. But the windows always remained covered. Still, to this day too.

* * * * *

The summer churned on, and finally it was July 14, 1974, my sixteenth birthday, which fell on a Sunday that year. After the usual routine of mass followed by a big homemade meal of meatloaf and mashed potatoes back at the house, I received my customary birthday lecture from my father, a surprisingly lighthearted one, as I recall, and we cut into the vanilla-frosted angel food cake my mother had made for me. Not long after that, Dad left without giving a reason. I sprawled on the couch and fell asleep until the sound of his return awakened me.

"Joe, come outside. I have something for you," he said.

I gave him a puzzled look and then glanced at Mom to see if she knew what was going on. She was smiling. We headed outside—Paul was on one of his walks—to the most beautiful thing a teenage boy could imagine: a red 1964 Plymouth Sport Fury with push-button automatic transmission and silver trim on both sides that Dad had bought from Aunt Lorena for $250. I was speechless. My father beamed, and Mom was almost giggling. Both were as happy as I had seen them in some time. I didn't know if the car was for my turning sixteen or to assuage their guilt for what had happened earlier in the summer with Paul, but either way, I was happy too. My days of walking to school were over. The Fury gave me freedom. I was soon able to get a job in the circulation department at the local *Guthrie Daily Leader*. I was responsible for filling the gas tank of my new car—and was able to escape the strained atmosphere of home since Paul had returned, as well as Paul himself.

Yes, I was avoiding my big brother. I knew my parents were aware of that, and I could sense the guilt they felt about the change in our family dynamics. Yet my relationship with Mom and Dad seemed to become closer for having shared the struggle to help Paul. Still, the incident with the knife earlier that summer had probably ensured that Paul's days in Guthrie were numbered. Paul soon announced that he would be moving back to Tulsa but not as a practicing priest.

My brother then went to work as a gas station attendant/salesman at Consumers Oil in Tulsa in January 1975, working fifty-four hours a week for $2.10 an hour. The still-young man who had never wanted or cared to work with his hands or get dirty was now changing oil, doing lube jobs, and selling batteries, tires, and car accessories. Paul became good at it too, according to our cousin Arlene, who said his boss had told her that "Paul was a really good worker." The man eventually promoted Paul to assistant manager at $2.50 an hour.

Paul worked at the station for two years but not without incident. By then, Arlene said, "[you] could tell he was sick." One of his coworkers either took notice or found reason to say or do something to Paul that did not sit right with my brother.

"Don't do it again," Paul supposedly dared the boy.

When the kid persisted, Paul grabbed him by the shoulders and lifted him into the air, saying, "I told you to never do that again!"

"The boy never did it again," Arlene said.

In future job applications, Paul would simply write "sickness" as his reason for leaving his job at the gas station. Dad was also right that Paul's being away on his own wouldn't last. After a few months of being unemployed, after giving away what money he had again and having no money for rent or food, Paul moved back home. More than a year later, in April 1978, he went to work with Dad, who had retired to build homes and furniture and teach carpentry at the Guthrie Job Corps.

Paul's new job as a carpenter's helper paid better than the gas station job had: He started at three dollars an hour and eventually made almost four. He also worked an eight-to-five workweek for the first time since becoming a priest.

At the time, I wasn't too far away, attending Central State University, about twenty minutes down the highway in Edmond, Oklahoma. To help pay for college, I had sold my Fury. Dad again haggled for me, getting $450 for the car, quite a profit back then.

The distance from home was just enough for me to escape the shadow cast by Paul after his return. And I flourished at CSU. A natural joiner and doer, I was busy there, between my studies and participating in such organizations as the Baptist Student Union, where one fellow student informed me that I was going to hell because I was

Catholic. The pace of university life left me with no time to think, much less worry, about how my parents were faring back in Guthrie with their oldest son back at home. They were left to endure the shadow every day.

* * * * *

Anyone who has had a close family member or friend with mental illness knows that you are always waiting for the next incident, the next rejection, the next heartbreak. Life will just have become ordered and fallen into a routine, maybe pleasant or not, and then *Bam*!—something will happen. In 1978, that something was not only unexpected but bizarre. Three months after Paul began to work with Dad, he left his job as a carpenter's helper to "reenter the Catholic priesthood." Paul would list the reason just like that on all future job applications.

The Reverend Eusebius J. Beltran had recently been ordained as the bishop of the Tulsa Diocese. Born in 1934, in Ashley, Pennsylvania, the fifth of eight children, Beltran was the son of a Spanish immigrant coal miner who died from black lung disease. Beltran had been ordained in Atlanta, Georgia, in 1960. Five years later, he marched in the Selma, Alabama, civil rights protest despite his archbishop warning Beltran and three other priests that he would not bail them out if they were arrested at the march. They marched anyway.

Beltran is a fairly short man with a low, soothing, sometimes monotone voice. He carefully thinks about and chooses his words, occasionally pausing to consider what he will say next. He was not one who ever aspired to be a bishop, but out of obedience and when asked, he became one. As a young bishop, he had overseen the tumultuous, previous decade post–Vatican II. He still faced a growing exodus of priests that threatened to cause a painful shortage. "Finding ones like Paul [out of the priesthood] was not unusual," Beltran said.

What was different in Paul's situation was the recent handwritten request Beltran had received from Paul:

I want to return to the priesthood. I want to be an active minister again.

Beltran followed up on that request with Paul. When they met, the former priest towered over the bishop, but Beltran said he liked and admired Paul at once. He knew Paul had lived "a life of the poor and gave his money away."

Beltran gave serious consideration to Paul's request and let Paul know that. Paul was elated, as shown in a May 15 handwritten letter.

> *Dear Bishop Beltran,*
>
> *Thank you for being so kind and helpful to me. Because of you I am full of confidence for the future, now I know Jesus wants me, really wants me to share in His priestly ministry and I am sure that He will provide the means to do so.*
>
> *As yet I am not certain I will be formally reinstated, this is, as you said, up to Church.*
>
> *I only want to have the certainty of doing God's will for that is the source of real and lasting joy.*
>
> *For helping me in this endeavor, thank you.*
>
> *Love,*
>
> *Paul Hight*

In May 1978, the diocese took the extraordinary step of seeking authorization for my brother's possible reinstatement from the Apostolic Nunciature, the diplomatic mission of the Holy See to the United States in Washington, D.C. A June 1 reply stated that the bishop would need to "make a detailed presentation" to the Sacred Congregation for the Clergy. Beltran informed Paul in a June 12, 1978, letter sent to our Guthrie home that he wanted to meet with him in ten days. With regard to "your request for reinstatement in the active priesthood," he added. "Where there is a possibility, there would be certain conditions and positive requirements."

JOE HIGHT

Beltran then sought input from other priests in the diocese. Dr. Inbody submitted a psychiatric report by October of that year. Father Dorney submitted a memorandum regarding a possible car and salary for Paul. He also called Paul.

By September, Paul had sent another handwritten letter from our Guthrie home, this time to Dorney:

> *Dear Denni,*
>
> *Thank you very much for your kindness to me. Even if I can't make it back as a priest, it will always be remembered.*
>
> *When you're in a situation like mine, it is easy to become discouraged at delays when you're uncertain about your whole future.*
>
> *It is good to have a friend like yourself who knows what to do, or if He doesn't find out very quickly, you are certainly in the right position.*
>
> *God will certainly bless you.*
>
> *Love,*
> *Paul Hight*

Then, just after Thanksgiving, the remote possibility seemed possible. On November 28, Paul, Bishop Beltran, and two witnesses signed a "growth plan agreement." Beltran had not gone into this blindly; he knew about Paul's past mental health issues. He would say they were evident when he met Paul. But Beltran had also never seen an official letter requesting Paul's laicization, but that didn't matter. He would still have to overturn a previous bishop's decision.

"That would have been virtually impossible," Beltran said years later after he had become archbishop and then archbishop emeritus for Oklahoma. "Once you're laicized, the likelihood is minimal that you can return. It has happened, but it's almost impossible. Even today, it's virtually impossible for those with mental illness to return."

"I felt he was a kind, good man," Beltran added. "It's the recognition . . ." His voice trailed off. He paused for almost a minute as if troubled by the words that followed. ". . . that a man can be a good person, but he's not fit for a ministry." Monsignor Dorney echoed Beltran's reasoning: ". . . the issue that he was laicized in the first place would be the reason for him not to be reinstated."

For those who believed Paul should still be a priest, whether in active ministry or not, his attempt to return to the priesthood was further proof that Paul had not wanted to leave the priesthood in the first place. As other priests would say later more than once, Paul believed he was a priest for life. The Catholic Church, however, did not want someone with severe mental illness among the brotherhood of priests.

It was as simple as that.

Paul's hope of becoming a priest evaporated in 1978. The Catholic Church he loved had rejected his request to return to the priesthood.

He rarely ever spoke about losing that life again.

He had to start over.

Chapter 11

Edging into Insanity

Paul perched on the edge of his bed in Hope Hall, Ward 31-D, Central State Griffin Memorial Hospital, Norman, Oklahoma. He had been committed to Oklahoma's hospital for the insane.

From the outside, however, with its white columns and ornate gates, its appearance could have led one to think that Paul was on a little respite, a trip to a resort even. Griffin did look more hotel than hospital, with its Mason & Hamlin grand piano and tranquil sitting area. Built in 1893, the building had housed a women's college before being sold to the Oklahoma Sanitarium Co. in 1895 with the objective of turning it into a mental health facility for the "violent insane." That mission proudly graced the facility's front entrance until 1899, when sanitarium officials hired psychiatrist David W. Griffin of North Carolina, who took one look at the word *insane* and took it upon himself to chisel it off. Griffin would become superintendent of the former Norman Institution for Violent Insane in 1902, a position he held until 1950.

Seven years later, a 1909 report by the Oklahoma social reformer Kate Barnard, then commissioner of charities and corrections, would refer to it as "the Norman insane asylum." In that year, 954 people were committed for twenty reasons that, as recorded, included hereditary insanity, ill health, imbeciles, epilepsy, old age, mental worry, inebriates, syphilis, idiots, overwork, privation (being deprived of food, money or basic rights), criminally insane, childbirth, injury to brain, self-abuse, sunstroke, and pellagra (a nutritional disorder stemming from a niacin deficiency, once known as Austrian leprosy).

By 1915, the Oklahoma Legislature had passed the "Lunacy Bill" creating asylums in towns such as Vinita, Fort Supply, and Norman. Paul would spend nearly a year in the Vinita and Norman facilities. The Norman site became Central State Hospital, but in a sign that attitudes had not changed all that much when it came to people with mental illness, many accounts can be found referring to it as "Central State Hospital for the Insane." At its peak in the early 1950s, Central State housed 1,500 to 3,600 people who had been committed voluntarily or by a court. The patients lived and worked on a 240-acre campus with large vegetable gardens, chicken houses, a hog farm, a dairy farm, a laundry, a bakery, a cannery, and power and ice plants, as well as a chapel and cemetery, in which those deemed insane and without family or those shunned by family were buried. A common grave elsewhere on the acreage held thirty-eight people killed in a fire at the hospital in the early hours of April 13, 1918.

In 1953, the place was renamed Central State Griffin Memorial Hospital for the man who had guided it since before the turn of the century. The Sixties were seven years away by then. Medical approaches to mental illness and standards of care for those with mental illness would start to evolve, but in 1950s Oklahoma, old prejudices about mental illness endured. In that decade, the state Department of Mental Health hired the University of Oklahoma to produce the video drama *Mental Hospital*. The main character of the short film is a patient named Fred Clanton, committed to the hospital by court order. Everything is dark, even the sky, as the film opens and Fred laments.

Oh my God, oh no, don't let them take me in there.
What will happen to me now?

A narrator in a deep, ominous voice echoes Fred's concerns:

> What will happen to Fred now? What happens to
> all of them—the men and women from all walks of life?

The video opens on a scene of people—some sad, some keeping to themselves, some laughing hysterically—as the narrator explains:

> Some patients are disturbed, unable to care for
> themselves in normal life situations. Others are physi-
> cally as well as mentally ill. Many are capable of limited
> adjustment, able to work at varied tasks within the hos-
> pital. . . . Deterioration. Chronic conditions, limited
> hope for some. Others may go home tomorrow.
>   Meanwhile, they are living here, 3,200 men and
> women all gathered together in a modern mental insti-
> tution, a city in itself, complete with every facility for
> effective treatment. . . . Patients are secure and comfort-
> able, and most of them are happy.

The nineteen-minute film seems to portray the "hospital for the insane" as a pleasant resort or retreat. It points out that patients can fish in the nearby lakes and work on the hospital farm so that those with rural backgrounds can "feel right at home." At Christmastime, Norman residents drive through the grounds to take in the light show, and in fair weather, locals picnic on the hospital grounds with the residents. The narrator goes on to explain who these residents are:

> They come from all sorts of homes, all sorts of back-
> grounds, but at somewhere along the line, life became
> too much for them.

Fred, it seems, believes everyone is out to get him, including his wife, Betty. The character undergoes various diagnoses and treatments, including a spinal tap. He is diagnosed with schizophrenia, paranoid type, the same eventual diagnosis that Paul received. But in 2019, some people watching the film might be disturbed by the treatments that Fred receives—insulin shock therapy and reinforced shock treatment, while other "disturbed patients" are strapped down on gurneys and treated with electroshock therapy, hydrotherapy, and sedative packs. Through it all, the narrator reminds us:

> The effective mental hospital must always serve as a refuge for its patients, a place where they can live quietly during that period of reorientation in which they learn how to achieve a better adjustment to that world outside.

The video points out that some patients never adjust, as a woman twirls with a scarf. Some show a complete loss of contact with reality, dark shadows across disordered minds. The character Fred, however, is recovering. He's shown drawing, watching movies, playing dominoes and pool, and dancing with women who are not Betty. He gets a job with the ground crew, working and sweating outside in the hot Oklahoma sun. Just before his release, he is seen smoking a cigarette with a "steady hand." The narrator proudly observes:

> How well he looks. A man can be proud of the things that he's created with his own two hands, and a hospital can be proud too. Proud to see a patient face the world as a man again.

The short film ends with Fred released after a six-month stay at the mental hospital. As Fred departs, he is seen looking longingly out the back window of a car at the place that has given his life back to him. He admits he was sick, *but now I am well, and I know it. I'm able to face the world again.* The implication is that that includes his own hometown, somewhere in Oklahoma, somewhere where he knows *I'll still face people who will stare, talk, and sneer.*

From what I know of my brother Paul's battle with mental illness, that old video is an oversimplification at best, alluding to a happy ending that many people with mental illness never get. My brother certainly didn't. Society's approach to mental illness has historically been a poor patchwork of care, especially in how people with mental illness are perceived and treated. In the eighteenth century, mental illness was generally treated as a physical illness, like a broken leg, until some people came to see it an illness of morality, a condition to be treated with humane care and a dose of strict moral discipline.

In a 2014 article in the journal *Cell*, Dr. John Krystal, a Yale professor and leading expert in schizophrenia and depression, observed of the 1700s, "Despite its limitations, its respectful treatment of people with mental illness and its efforts to meet the basic needs of people, albeit through asylums, had a transformative impact in Western Europe."

The idea of humane treatment for people with mental illness was an improvement over the use of bleeding, purging, and vomiting championed in the 1600s. Or the low blood sugar comas of the 1930s (a treatment that didn't fall from favor until the 1960s). Or the inducing of seizures, which was allowed until 1982, as well as treatments such as exorcism, ice water baths, the use of chains and shackles (common prior to the 1950s). And lobotomies, which won its inventor Egas Moniz the 1949 Nobel Prize but was soon seen as too ineffective to warrant the dangers that came with them except in a few specific diagnoses.

My brother arrived at Griffin during a new societal approach to the care of people with mental illness: No longer would people be locked up in institutions. Instead, they would be free to live with family, in group homes, or on their own if their illness allowed. What followed was a massive deinstitutionalization effort that continued into the 1980s and some people would say continues to this day. The 1970s saw the number of patients housed at Griffin go from some 3,000 patients to as low as 300 patients at times; by 1990, 245 patients remained. At the end of 2018, patient capacity was 120, and stays were measured in weeks or days, not months, years, or a lifetime. The once thriving institution, the minicity, had become a temporary stopover for Oklahomans struggling with mental illness and was fast on its way to being considered a blight and embarrassment to the nearby university community in Norman. As one resident of the city observed, "Griffin is creepy. I try to turn my head every time I drive past it."

* * * * *

Paul's diagnosis on arrival at the Norman hospital had been "schizophrenia, catatonic type." His prognosis: "guarded."

"Patient was brought to Central State Hospital by his father because has been in a catatonic stupor during the past few days and has had sudden blurring of vision," a release summary of Paul's "voluntary" admission read. "[Patient] was very confused on admission."

Inside Ward 31-D, Paul found conditions more akin to those depicted in the 1975 film *One Flew over the Cuckoo's Nest* than the images shared in the 1950s feel-good *Mental Hospital* film. If he stood, he nearly hit his head on the low ceiling. If he looked outside, he most likely saw the side of another building. If he went barefoot, he walked on sanded rock floors. He shared a room with seven to eight other men behind a steel door, shorter than he was, with a slit cut in the metal so attendants could look in as needed.

Each ward had a larger dayroom at the end of the hallway where residents could escape their crowded, barricaded rooms during specified times. The room's only diversion for the patients, beyond conversation, was a small black-and-white television that remained on the same channel for hours at a time. With no air-conditioning during the summer, the hospital became a hot, sweaty place that smelled of mildew and urine. For those who had permission, there was also a screened porch, the screens being there to prevent anyone from jumping or escaping.

One of the common sayings shared by those who have spent time at Griffin is, "If you're not crazy when you enter Griffin, you're crazy when coming out of it." Living there was not something easily forgotten. One former patient who was committed there but released many years ago admitted to still feeling a pang of anxiety just hearing the name. "They treated us like animals," she told friends. "The sounds at night were people yelling or people being mistreated."

Paul would return five times to Griffin, as did another man, Jerry Dan "J. R." Risenhoover. As Paul had, Risenhoover grew to dread the return. First admitted in 1964 at the age of twenty-one, he recalled before his death in April 2018 that his parents had delivered him to Griffin the first time. Four more times would follow, the last in 2007, despite his having been misdiagnosed as "paranoid schizophrenic" the first time. Risenhoover was a manic depressive with a bipolar disorder.

Risenhoover went on to work thirty-four years as a psychiatric social worker at state facilities throughout Oklahoma, so he has seen the inside as both patient and employee. He repeatedly described Griffin Memorial as "terrible." Despite it having been more than a decade since Risenhoover was last committed to Griffin Memorial, the man stuttered with emotion and had to take multiple breaks as he shared what he had witnessed and experienced at the hospital. He spoke of patients being forced to sleep on the floor and being put in a room with a patient who had spread his feces all over the room. No staffer ever came to clean up the mess, and living and dealing with the feces became Risenhoover's new normal. "They would put you in the room, and you would have to fend for yourself," he said.

Risenhoover explained why that sometimes turned deadly. After the mother of a twenty-year-old blind woman named Courtney placed her daughter in Griffin Memorial, the young woman was allowed to wander outside without supervision. On one such walk, she ended up in a nearby pond and drowned. Hers was an unnecessary death. Risenhoover said, "It was quite a blow to her mother—she went to pieces." As for Risenhoover, he was eventually put on lithium, which is now known to cause problems with the kidneys, although if caught early in treatment, the kidney damage can be reversed. Risenhoover was not so lucky. He ended up with permanent kidney damage that required a kidney transplant.

By her count, Linda K. Kerr was committed to Griffin Memorial a "record sixty-five times" from 1976 to 2014. Well educated like Paul, with a master's degree, she received a similar diagnosis as Risenhoover finally did: bipolar, Type 1 manic depressive, and fell into an unhealthy cycle. The court would commit her, Griffin would put her on medication, and then Griffin would release her. When Kerr was on her own on the outside, her behavior followed a predictable downward spiral: She would quit taking her medication and start making poor decisions. She wouldn't sleep. Wouldn't eat. Wouldn't stop shopping. And she would party too much.

Kerr was committed for the first time in 1967. She was twenty-one. A second commitment followed that same year. She described the conditions and treatment at Griffin Memorial as "horrible." At one point, sixty women shared a room. Kerr recalled a young woman becoming too loud one day so "a three-hundred-pound staff member came in and sat on her—and expelled gas on her."

As Risenhoover had, Kerr remembered someone dying unnecessarily at Griffin, a different someone. The middle-aged woman was sleeping not two feet from Kerr when she woke moaning and unable to get up. The attendants came in and rolled the woman off the bed and onto the floor. They did not seek medical attention for her. The woman died of a complication that stemmed from being unable to have a bowel movement. Kerr had no memory of staff showing any interest or remorse at the time. "There are so many sob, sad stories," she said. ". . . I have many friends who did not make it."

Kerr herself spent days alone, strapped on a metal bed, in one of what she called three "dungeon . . . jail cell" rooms in the back of Building 5. Her wrists, waist, and ankles were constrained with thick leather belts. Attendants would tilt the bed up to feed her and then leave, often failing to have provided a bathroom break. In response to this, some patients took to rubbing their feces on the walls. Staff members had to repeatedly repaint the room to hide the marks patients had scratched into the concrete with their fingernails. And then there were the two Native American women placed in cells on either side of Kerr's; the women screamed day and night. "War cries," Kerr called it. She came to sympathize with their primal screams. Later, after being strapped down in the dungeon again on another day, Kerr was moved to screams herself. " 'This is hell!' " Kerr said she screamed. " 'Let me die, God! Let me die!' "

Her prayer that day wasn't answered, but Kerr did hear God tell her to be baptized and saved. Her conversion that day saved her life, she said. She went from taking sixteen medications a day to eating healthy. Recovered now, she exudes the enthusiasm of a born-again preacher. And if you cross her path, you can be assured she will ask you whether or not you've been saved.

* * * * *

The first floor of Griffin Memorial had its grand piano, but the second floor of Hope Hall housed a surgery wing and dental clinic for Oklahoma inmates. Thus, those deemed insane shared their building with those deemed criminal. At Griffin Memorial, if a patient misbehaved or was perceived to have misbehaved, the patient was placed in a "comfort room" with low light and a mattress until the patient settled down. If the patient was violent or a threat to self, the patient was stripped naked and placed in mechanical restraints on a bed in the "seclusion room." That room was painted a dull white when Paul first arrived. Later, staff members would scrawl a peace symbol and the words "love, joy and happiness" on the walls.

Between 1976 and 1991, Paul spent at least 242 days in treatment centers or mental institutions in Oklahoma, with most of the time either at Griffin Memorial or Eastern State. Records indicate he also might have spent an additional six months or more in either Hillcrest or Saint Francis hospitals in Tulsa or crisis centers in Tulsa or Oklahoma City. Would he have been in any of those treatment centers or mental institutions longer, maybe long enough to truly get well, if deinstitutionalization hadn't become the standard by the time Paul became a part of system? We will never know.

In Oklahoma, county sheriffs had to drive those deemed as suffering from mental illness or having a mental disorder to Central State or a metropolitan crisis center. Rural areas, even those not far from a big city, lacked the capacity to deal with residents going through psychotic episodes. In some instances, law-enforcement officers would give a one-way bus ticket to particularly troubling residents so they could get to a metro area and receive the services or treatment they needed. As it had been since the 1950s, Central State was often a dumping place for such people. Some people never returned home, opting to remain in the metropolitan areas, either in low-rent subsidized housing or on the streets. Others, such as Paul, went back and forth to family. Some were veterans. Some had been rejected by their own families and become homeless.

Most were impacted by deinstitutionalization, which was building momentum at the time. Instead of spending months or years in, say, Griffin Memorial, people stayed for a few days or a few weeks before being sent back into the community, with occasional follow-ups treated at specialized clinics. But for many, even those shorter periods of hospitalization seemed too long, and that led to the 1963 Community Mental Health Centers Act. Created during the freewheeling Sixties, the act was intended to provide people who suffered from severe mental illness with more independence and an improved quality of life in the community in which they lived. The introduction of antipsychotic drugs in the 1950s had allowed more people with severe mental illness to remain living on their own or with family. The 1963 act provided federal funds to begin to build treatment care centers in communities to support that. However, the act was never fully funded and created unintended consequences.

According to the report Deinstitutionalization: Its Impact on Community Mental Health Centers and the Seriously Mentally Ill:

> The individuals who were to receive the benefits of deinstitutionalization were often homeless, isolated, and victimized. Some individuals with SMI who were released from institutions deteriorated, were reinstitutionalized, and some lost their lives.

By 1977, 650 community health centers were treating some 1.9 million patients with diagnosed mental illness a year, and law enforcement was often involved when those same patients showed signs of their illness. Three years later, President Jimmy Carter signed the Mental Health Systems Act, which sought to restructure the community mental health system and improve services for those with severe mental illness. Yet only one year later under President Ronald Reagan, the government ended its role as a service provider to the mentally ill, opting instead to send block grants to the states. To this day, many mental health advocates blame Reagan for creating widespread issues for people who suffered from mental illness as well as their families and communities.

The New York Times addressed the issue twice in editorials. In 1981, it called deinstitutionalization "a cruel embarrassment, a reform gone terribly wrong." In 1984, it stated, "The policy that leads to the release of most of the nation's mentally ill patients from the hospital to the community is now regarded as a major failure."

When Paul had a psychotic episode, he would usually return to Central State, but under the new standards, we never knew when he would be released back into the community. What was relatively easy to see was when it was time for Paul to be in an institution again. On his medication and doing well, Paul was friendly and welcoming with people. Off his medication and doing poorly, he could be sullen and agitated, sometimes even giddy, because of what the voices in his head were saying. The voices often began by telling Paul that he was fine and did not need his medication, which was labeled as "chemotherapy" on some of his records. Other times, Paul would grow weary of the side effects of the medication, which for him could be dramatic, enough to make him nervous around anyone. He would become more brazen with where he smoked, and soon Dad would be driving Paul back to Norman.

No rule in canon law forbids priests from smoking, and in the 1960s, smoking widely accepted in this country and in seminaries, with an estimated 42 percent of Americans regular smokers, according to the Population Reference Bureau. So although the start of Paul's smoking habit might remain in question, there is little doubt that his habit was exacerbated by his time spent in mental health facilities. During the 1980s and 1990s, industry documents show that tobacco companies targeted psychiatric facilities, providing free cigarettes by the hundreds to hospitals and marketing cigarettes to patients with schizophrenia. The facilities also requested cigarette donations. Staff members rewarded patients with cigarettes for taking their medication or gave them smoke breaks for good behavior. As a result, one in three adults with mental illness smoke compared to one in five adults without mental illness, and roughly 40 percent of cigarettes sold in the United States are smoked by people with mental health issues ranging from depression and anxiety to substance-abuse problems.

Studies also show that people with mental illness who smoke die about five years earlier than those without mental health issues. Such statistics left psychologists torn between the positive, calming effects of smoking and the dire health effects of cigarettes. Some were supportive of patients who smoked excessively. Attendants also smoked at a higher rate, and some of them encouraged patients to smoke as a way to self-medicate. A 2006 study found 65 percent to 85 percent of patients smoked. In more recent years, however, many psychiatrists and therapists have come to believe that quitting smoking helps people's mental condition. Given that people with serious mental illness treated in the public health system die twenty-five years earlier than those without mental illness, many doctors and therapists now counsel their patients not to add the risk of smoking.

Risenhoover's parents had taught him not to smoke or drink, but he recalled being constantly pressured to smoke at Griffin Memorial. Attendants and other patients would hand him lighted cigarettes. He remembers patients being rewarded with cigarettes for good behavior.

"Everybody smoked. It was the thing to do," he said.

That seems foolhardy in retrospect. With the death rate for people with mental illness so high, Paul already faced a likely early death—smoking raised that risk considerably. Yet Paul never stopped. His smoking addiction continued for the rest of his life. Everywhere he lived, anything he had touched always reeked of cigarettes.

When Paul was off his medication, his behavior would become more and more erratic and the voices more insistent, and soon he would end up committed to a crisis center for initial diagnosis, and then it was on to a mental institution. That was the pattern until the early 1990s when, for unknown reasons, the commitments suddenly stopped, even though he continued to have psychotic episodes.

The process of committing Paul would start with a phone call, usually from the sheriff, a mental health clinic, or supervisor at work to Dad. "Do you want us to take him to the crisis center?" Sheriff J. C. Burris would say. The answer was usually yes.

A big, burly, and considerate man, Sheriff Burris was the state's first elected black county sheriff. I later worked with him on my first job after college as a reporter for the *Guthrie Daily Leader*. The paper had an agreement with the sheriff. He would call us when there was any incident: Murders. Suicides. Oil-field accidents. Early morning. The middle of a hot afternoon. Late at night. It didn't matter. Sheriff Burris always called. He would do the same with my parents when anything happened with Paul.

However, the first time Paul was brought to Central State Griffin Memorial Hospital, the hospitalization wasn't triggered by a call from the sheriff. In December 1976, a thirty-three-year-old Paul had fallen into a catatonic state from staring at the sun. He was living away from home at the time, working at the Tulsa gas station. His vision suddenly blurred, and someone called our father. Dad drove the ninety-five miles to Tulsa, picked Paul up, and then drove another 125 miles to Central State Hospital. The admission this time was voluntary.

"Father states [his son] hears voices, has been in a catatonic stupor," the treatment plan and progress notes read.

Daily logs tracked Paul's progress or lack of it. He said the voices caused him to go into a catatonic stupor. When family members visited him, Paul talked about hearing voices or about his interactions with the devil. Logs show Paul was also having "auditory hallucinations, withdrawn behavior, insomnia." My brother spent time in the comfort and seclusion rooms too, according to the logs, because he was "hostile at intervals." Later, when he was stabilized, attendants encouraged him to get off his bed and become more social in the ward.

It was during this time that Paul made clear he planned to return to Tulsa and revealed for the first time that he had a girlfriend, even though he was still considering a plea to return to the priesthood. The woman's name was Janet Lynne Brown; Paul called her Lynne. A nurse, she had been one of the people who cared for him during the times he had been placed earlier in Saint Francis Hospital. That was all he said about Lynne that day. Maybe he was conflicted about having a girlfriend while also thinking about returning to the priesthood.

The first time he was committed, Paul spent only eight days at Griffin Memorial before being discharged a week before Christmas. Doctors encouraged him to take his medication, five milligrams of the antipsychotic Stelazine, and to join a medication group at Tulsa Mental Health Clinic.

"Patient is ambulatory, conscious, coherent, cooperative, in good contact with surroundings," his release summary signed by Drs. A. B. Danesh and F. P. Hebron stated. "He denies having delusions, hallucinations, or suicidal thought, much better now."

"Much better now" seems overly optimistic in retrospect, considering Paul's history in the 1970s, but nonetheless, he returned to Tulsa for a little longer. The confrontation with his fellow worker at the gas station would be one of several altercations while Paul was off his medication. Another at the beginning of the next decade would be among the most bizarre incidents involving my brother.

It would cause Paul to deny his own identity and send him to the "hospital for the criminally insane."

Chapter 12

Home of the Criminally Insane

A tall, hulking man in his late thirties, looking disheveled and reeking of cigarette smoke, walked into a Tulsa hotel.

"I own this Holiday Inn and every Holiday Inn in the universe," he announced loudly.

A stunned clerk said, "Uh, sir, can I help you?"

"I own this Holiday Inn!"

"Who are you?"

"Adolf Hitler!"

The man was unemployed and living somewhere in Tulsa. He might have been wandering the streets and digging into trash cans for food. He was agitated when he stomped into the Holiday Inn in downtown Tulsa. Why the man decided to visit this Holiday Inn on this January day in 1980 is unknown; it just might have been the one closest to him. The weather was warm for the time of year, a high of 50 degrees Fahrenheit—warm enough for anyone to roam the streets.

A Holiday Inn manager confronted the man. A scuffle ensued. A hotel employee called the Tulsa Police Department, and police came and arrested the man on an assault and battery complaint and took him to the Tulsa Municipal Jail. Police must have found a wallet on "Hitler," because they soon identified him as thirty-eight-year-old Paul Wilber Hight. His new self-bestowed moniker was as unlike the Paul that his family and friends knew as it could be. As a child of a World War II veteran and then as a priest, Paul had despised the acts of the German Third Reich. Yet as an ill man who could be controlled by voices, he became this night not only its infamous leader but also the owner of every Holiday Inn in the universe, according to him.

At his district court hearing, the judge asked Paul who he was and if he had a spouse, a father, a mother, or any next of kin. My brother replied that he did not, and a clerk wrote "unk.," meaning "unknown," on the court document. A public defender asked again who he was.

"I'm Adolf Hitler."

The judge asked what he was doing in the hotel.

"I own all of the Holiday Inns in the universe."

The court document noted, "Subject may be a danger to himself or others."

Two days later, at 9:30 a.m., January 30, 1980, a judge in Tulsa District Court ordered Paul's continued detainment. Tulsa County District Judge M. M. McDougal issued the order using "provisions of Sections 54 and 55 of the Mental Health Law of 1953" that allowed for involuntary detention of a person suffering from mental illness.

> . . . It appearing to the court . . . and after a full investigation of said matter (without) the verdict of a jury that said person is a person requiring treatment and should be admitted to a medical facility as a patient; that all of the laws of the State of Oklahoma have been complied with, and there is no less restrictive appropriate treatment available.

In layman's terms, Paul would be taken to Eastern State Hospital in Vinita "under a detention order which was subsequently changed to court certification . . ."

By then, authorities had identified Paul as a former priest who had twenty years of education, but for some reason, they listed him as having been unemployed for five years. Documents include his parents' names but show their birthplaces as "unknown." Paul's place of birth is listed as "Oklahoma," but his last known residence, as "like."

A line in the "What Relatives Have had Mental or Nervous Trouble" section toward the bottom of the document state: "Grandmother committed suicide." Odd given that Grandma Kingston had suffered from dementia or Alzheimer's and died of old age. Grandma Hight had died of old age too, although her smoking habit likely accelerated her death. Neither grandmother had killed herself. The next day, Paul was taken to Eastern State, or the home of the criminally insane, as it had become known. And oddly, he was not taken there by the police or the sheriff but by Father Dennis Dorney.

The state of Oklahoma used the Vinita facility as a treatment center for inmates and all court-ordered observations and evaluations. Paul was placed there even though this was the first time he had been charged with an actual crime. He was among hundreds of people with mental illness sent there. According to a study prepared for the Oklahoma Department of Mental Health, courts ordered 257 men and 24 women to be determined competent or incompetent at Eastern State from March 1, 1978, to February 28, 1979, less than a year after a judge sent Paul there. Of those, two hundred men and seventeen women were found competent while forty-one men and five women were found incompetent, 16 percent of those were detained.

Vinita is about sixty-five miles northeast of Tulsa, with a population that has hovered under six thousand for years. The town is the birthplace of TV personality *Dr. Phil* McGraw and home to what has long been known as the world's largest McDonald's, an arched glass restaurant that spans Interstate 44. Built as a service plaza in 1957, before it became a McDonald's, it is a popular stopping place for tourists. The more infamous site in Vinita, however, might well be Eastern State Hospital, now surrounded by a fence topped with barbed wire. An Oklahoma City TV report would one day proclaim, "The vast majority of Oklahomans with mental illness will never commit a crime. However, those who do often end up being the most bizarre, horrific type of criminal." Like Central State in Norman, the Vinita hospital has been around since the early days of statehood. Approved by the Oklahoma legislature in 1909, the hospital opened sixty-seven years before Paul's arrest. The first three hundred patients were shipped in on a special train from the Norman sanatorium and dropped off at Asylum Spur, more than a mile from the hospital. The patients either walked or rode in wagons the rest of the way. By 1954, the hospital was renamed Eastern State and became a minicity, not unlike Central State, with 2,800 people living there. Eastern State had a farm, one that featured some of the most prized Holstein dairy cattle in the state, along with seventy-five wards and 460 employees. The hospital also had a cemetery.

By the time Paul arrived in 1980, with deinstitutionalization in full swing, the eighteen wards housed fewer than four hundred residents. The average length of stay was a little more than a month. Paul would stay for more than three-and-a-half months. As with Central State, Eastern State's appearance was deceiving; the place could have been mistaken for a red-brick apartment complex.

Visitation rules were strict.

1. No smoking.
2. No food item or clothing article of any kind.
3. Absolutely no misconduct.
4. If rules are broken, rights to visitation of any kind will be lost.

Taking photographs was prohibited too.

Some rooms had an open steel toilet, not unlike ones found in a prison cell. Other rooms had a communal bathroom with a rule that patients had to be attended by staff at all times, and shower-room doors must be kept closed. Long, tiled hallways led to the rooms. A welcome sign provided the date, when the next holiday was, the season, and the weather of the day. Like Central State, Eastern State also had dental and medical facilities on site, as well as a library where patients could check out paperback books, magazines, and puzzles if they followed the rules. The hospital's amenities also included a canteen, beauty and barber shops, an auditorium that doubled as a gym, and All Faiths Chapel, which offered a worship service at 8:30 a.m. on Sundays and a Catholic Mass at 10 a.m. Tuesdays, which would not have fulfilled Paul's Sunday Mass obligation.

Doctors evaluated Paul on his arrival and found him to be "very delusional . . . and somewhat hostile when pressed." My brother was still claiming he was Hitler and owned all Holiday Inns. He denied knowing anyone else. Bob Adams, a nurse at the time, described Paul's condition in a long checklist: "disheveled, guarded, hostile, suspicious, withdrawn, bizarre, aggressive, disorganized," and thinking "ideas of unreality."

Treating such a condition was not an exact science, and the hospital tried to make that clear. They also tried to clarify up front, in the social history questionnaire the patients had to complete, the facility's objectives for the clients:

> Treatment for nervous or mental illness is different from other illnesses as its patient cannot be helped by medicine alone. . . . In mental illness, the doctor needs to know what ideas go through the patient's mind, how the patient felt about them, and how these ideas and feelings developed. Clues to these mental processes are given [to] the doctor by learning something about the patient's history: the kind of person the patient has been, how he felt toward the people around him, toward family and friends, what he talked about, and how he talked. The doctor measures improvement in the patient by knowing the kind of person he was before he became mentally ill.

A look at Paul's questionnaire shows many of the questions left unanswered. Father Dorney supplied answers to some questions, using the little he remembered, including that Paul liked "drama in college." Even though he couldn't recall this years later, Dorney also said on February 6, 1980, that "the Diocese of Tulsa has been providing (Paul) with a monthly support check." Another sparsely filled-out form in Paul's file contained a statement about my brother that my father would likely have agreed with, at least in part:

> [Patient] can live *normally* when he takes his medi-
> cation, but he refuses to take it regularly and thinks that
> he knows more than the doctor about proper dosage,
> etc. Even when on [medication], he tends to be rather
> lazy and does not want to take correction or suggestions.

On each document, red lettering stated, among other things, that "The Information disclosed may only be redisclosed to carry out the recipient's official duties with regard to the client's criminal proceeding. . . ." That document claimed the patient "believes he has unusual powers, believes he is influenced by supernatural forces or spirits, thinks others plan to harm him, hears voices, sees things," and "believes he is someone other than himself."

With the paperwork done, Paul was seen by three doctors, two staff physicians, and a psychologist. Their assessments echoed the nurse's that my brother suffered from significant psychological problems from the past and now had a history of psychiatric treatment. However, the doctors could not agree on whether Paul was suffering from both auditory and visual hallucinations.

Staff physician Dr. J. A. Nunez wrote:

> He believes he has unusual powers, also believes that
> because of those powers, he is influenced by the super-
> natural forces and spirits. . . . patient has no insight into
> his condition and showed little motivation for treatment.
> It should be noted that at times during the interview, he
> was suspicious, cautious, evasive, and guarded.

The second staff physician, Dr. V. N. Vadhawkar, wrote, "He has a long history of mental illness, and he has received previous treatment in different hospitals as well as with different psychiatrists. He was very delusional and had ideas of grandiosity and was having auditory and visual hallucinations." He then added: "He denied taking any illegal drugs or alcohol. Physically he was in good health." Psychologist Dr. Marion Sigurdson, however, wrote, "[Patient] stated he has auditory hallucinations, but he denied visual, gustatory, somatic, and olfactory hallucinations." In other words, Paul was hearing voices but not hallucinating. Sigurdson observed, "In general, the patient's thought content is autistic."

My father would later recall feeling somewhat bitter about Paul denying his own identity and the existence of a family that had never done anything, in Dad's eyes, but try to help this oldest child. As for the shock of my brother claiming to be Hitler, that would be a nightmare for any parent, much less one who had fought in World War II. Nonetheless, Dad accepted as inevitable that Paul would return home to Guthrie again—if only because regularly making the almost two-hundred mile, round trip to Vinita when Paul needed them was more than Dad and Mom could handle.

Eventually, all three doctors at Eastern State correctly diagnosed my brother. His medical record read: schizophrenia, paranoid type. The diagnosis would remain with Paul for the rest of his life. The doctors also put Paul on medication. They described it as "prescribed chemotherapeutic medication," and Paul's medical records show that the drug regimen eventually improved some of the mental health issues he was having, although also created new health problems. From the number of times the doctors prescribed the antacid Maalox—the records say, "repeatedly," the medications must have been eating away at his stomach.

Records also indicate that when doctors finally saw improvement in both Paul's mental and physical symptoms, they changed his medication from the antipsychotic drug Haldol to one hundred milligrams of the drug Mellaril, which treats schizophrenia specifically. The good news was that Mellaril, or thioridazine, did not upset his stomach; the bad news, the drug had numerous side effects. Meanwhile, Sigurdson recommended that Paul be hospitalized for a short period, "evaluated further, and then considered for referral to other therapeutic activities." That never happened. Yet in some ways Paul improved. He began to converse with his fellow patients and make friends. He was allowed to leave the building and move about the hospital grounds. He could take short trips home to Guthrie, trips that were deemed successful. Days and weeks passed, spring came, and soon his time at the hospital was being kept in months. My father talked to the doctors about releasing Paul so he could move home, saying he could help find Paul a part-time job and, with the help of Mom, provide the supervision Paul required. The request was not frivolous and the offer not lightly made. Dad and Mom knew Paul was not 100 percent.

An attendant at the time wrote, "Mr. Hight has improved. . . . Still says (he's) hearing voices now and then, but they are good voices and (he) doesn't mind hearing them." Dad seemed to believe Paul was well enough to safely live at home. Looking back, I can't help but wonder if Dad saw or chose to ignore a warning lurking in the attendant's report:

> [Patient] refused to take his medication. . . . He
> thinks that he knows better than the doctor.

Paul's stay at Eastern had triggered another problem: the end of any possible support by the Tulsa Diocese. No specific reason was given, but in a letter dated March 26, 1980, Father Dorney, acting as chancellor or in-house counsel for the Tulsa Diocese, had agreed to pay Paul's apartment rent. That correspondence would be the last from the diocese involving Paul.

Back in Vinita, in May 1980, some good news: Dr. Vadhawkar ruled Paul "well improved and . . . cooperating and . . . no problem on the ward. He was socializing with other patients and did not get violent or disturbed at any time and was not dangerous to himself or others."

Paul would be released. After being warned to take his medication regularly, visit an outpatient clinic in a month, and basically stay out of trouble, Paul was then released from Eastern State May 14, 1980. Doctors listed his condition as "prognosis guarded." He returned to Guthrie under the supervision of our parents. The Tulsa assault and battery charges were not pursued.

At the same time Paul was being released from Eastern State, I graduated from Central State University, now the University of Central Oklahoma, in a manner I could only hope made my parents proud. The student body had voted me outstanding senior man, and the journalism school had named me outstanding journalism graduate. Earlier in 1980, I had won a statewide investigative award for my reporting on The Way, a group described by *Encyclopedia Britannica* as a small religious cult that combines "Christian fundamentalism with Pentecostalism's emphasis on the supernatural gifts of the Holy Spirit." For the last four years, I had also worked at the college newspaper, *The Vista*, and ended as its editor, but at the time, the farthest I had ever traveled was to the Dallas area. I knew little about job prospects outside Oklahoma, and maybe, as a result, I would be returning home, as Paul would be, to Guthrie.

I had accepted a position on my hometown newspaper, the *Guthrie Daily Leader*, which was not exactly where I wanted to be. Paul was returning to work part time again for our father, something he probably didn't relish either. We would both be gone and on to other jobs in relative short order: I would move to Shawnee, Oklahoma, after refusing the *Leader*'s general manager's order to fire a reporter he didn't like. My brother to a new job working as a part-time flagman for $611 a month with the state highway department.

Paul fared well at the DOT, now the Oklahoma Department of Transportation, or ODOT. Within two months, ODOT hired him on full time with a pay raise to $781 a month, and then within a matter of days, they bumped him to $898 a month and gave him the official title of traffic service worker. For the first time in many years, Paul was making enough money to be independent again. He had a credit union and bank account. He renewed old friendships with people he had grown up with in Guthrie, made new ones with people who shared his interests, including in social justice, and struck up correspondences with like-minded friends who had moved away. In August of that year, a Speck Reynolds wrote to give Paul his new mailing address in Indiana, along with an update on how his own relocation was going.

> *We are members of Christ the King Parish. We attended the 8:30 a.m. Mass today, and we love the liturgy. Father gave a beautiful homily on forgiveness, and everyone participated in the kiss of peace. Hope everything is running smoothly for you. Love, Speck*

Could this Speck Reynolds have been the same Speck Reynolds whom *The Oklahoma Courier* identified in 1968 as a moderator of a panel about open housing in Edmond, an Oklahoma City suburb that would become notorious for being a haven for white flight, a "sundown town" where blacks were not welcome after dark? Edmond's Saint John the Baptist Catholic Church hosted the program, and one of the questions raised during it was whether blacks were welcomed in Edmond. Identified in the article as a Sunday school teacher at Saint John's, that Reynolds reportedly asked: "Is an all-white town with its all-white children, all-white schools, and all-white YMCA a breeding ground for racism?" The question was one I knew would have resonated with my brother, just as Reynolds's words about forgiveness in his letter must have.

Paul kept the letters he received from friends such as Reynolds for the rest of his days. Those that came during his difficult transition to secular life must have been particularly special to him because they meant he still had friends who cared enough about him to try to understand what he was going through.

He was now a transportation maintenance worker at ODOT, and his first job evaluation had yielded mostly satisfactory marks with an "above average" for cooperation and dependability. "Paul is very dependable and takes an interest in whatever job he is assigned. I consider him a real asset to our crew," wrote his supervisor, Garland Crabtree, a man whom Paul both liked and grew to respect and admire in his years with ODOT. ODOT's efforts before an upcoming snowstorm resulted in Paul making the Tuesday, February 2, 1982, *Guthrie Daily Leader*. A photo shows Paul in a jacket and hard hat with Crabtree and another worker, Raymond Sears. In typical Oklahoma fashion, the day's forecast called for gusty winds and temperatures hovering around 32 degrees Fahrenheit with fog, rain, and snow all on the same day. Such weather would keep or send most Oklahomans inside but not ODOT employees. Working in the state's fickle weather was a burden of the job, and so it was telling that whenever Paul was asked if he liked his job, he always said he liked Crabtree but hated—a word he rarely used—being on twenty-four-hour call in winter. Paul's mental illness had forced my highly educated brother into manual labor that, although it was good honest work, he was neither prepared for nor inclined to do. Ironically, however, his blue-collar job with ODOT did finally give Paul the validation that he had never received from the Catholic Church as a priest.

Nominated in January 1981, Paul was named "Maintenance Man of the Month" that May, with Crabtree writing Paul had shown good safety practices, helped with all types of maintenance, and was always prompt for work. "He has an excellent attitude and sense of humor. He gets along well with everyone," Crabtree wrote, adding that Paul was not only an asset to his crew but to "our district and the department." Paul's boss saw him as an asset to the crew, but the feeling might not have been universally shared by Paul's coworkers. Our brother Bill recalled Paul confiding to him: "The people there are mean and rude."

"He didn't like [his coworkers] too much," Bill said years later. "I think they realized that Paul was well educated, knew he had problems, and made fun of him."

Still, a job is a job, and sometimes a job is a needed routine, providing a steady, although perhaps paltry income and, thus a way to pay the bills and buy a little freedom. Paul's 1981 tax return shows he made $6,390.65. If he had worked a full year, he wrote in a job application, his annual salary would have been $11,315. In October of 1982, that salary allowed Paul to put down a $200 security deposit and agree to pay an adjusted rate of $184 a month to live in Apartment No. 10 of the

First Capitol Apartments in Guthrie. The complex had been built using grant money from the U.S. Department of Agriculture's Rural Rental Development Section 515 Rural Rental Housing Program. The Farmers Home Administration provided subsidies for low-income residents. Paul's apartment with 810 square feet rented for $305 a month, but the subsidy allowed him to pay 25 percent of his "adjusted monthly income" instead. He also received a $40 per month subsidy for paying his own utilities. For a man who had spent most of his life either sharing rooms, living in a hospital ward, or occupying what amounted to a monk's cell, the apartment must have seemed like a mansion. Whether it made Paul happy, that is difficult to know. I will never forget how much he loved that tiny, sparse bedroom that came with his first assignment as a priest.

With his medication keeping the voices either quiet, at bay, or bearable, Paul was slowly building himself a life not unlike a typical single man living on a budget. He bought a car, a 1975 Chevrolet Impala four-door sedan with only five thousand miles on it. He obtained a library card so he could read for free as much as he liked, his tastes running to books about the Catholic faith. Paul might no longer have been a Catholic priest, but he remained a steadfast Catholic, although at first, he rarely attended mass. That could have been because, as mentioned before, the Church frowned on and tried to forbid former priests from being in parish settings with people who knew they had once been a priest. When Paul did begin to attend mass in Guthrie, he no longer sat at the front of the church or in the old family pew or with our parents. Instead, he sat in the back, departing quickly afterward, before the socializing began.

At ODOT, Paul continued to do well. On his next performance review, Crabtree rated Paul above average in cooperation and dependability and above average in the quality of his work. Crabtree took time to note that Paul was getting along with his fellow crew members and the traveling public, once more calling my brother a "real asset to . . . the department." Unfortunately, this period of relative calm would be short-lived. By the end of the year, Paul was in court again—and wondering if the state highway department would give him a second chance.

Chapter 13

The Dreaded Phone Calls

The call came one evening, and I knew before I answered that it was my father. Dad was always the one who called with news of Paul. Dad's voice was calm but stern: "Joe, I have some bad news."

I had already braced myself—calls from my dad at this time of night were never good news; they usually meant Paul was off his meds again and in trouble. After a short pause, Dad bluntly said: "I've just come back from the doctor. I have cancer."

I managed to say, "What is it?"

". . . they think it's prostate cancer."

In the 1980s, prostate cancer was still a death sentence. My voice trembled as I said, "I'm sorry. What can I do?"

What I was trying to ask was what could we do to keep him alive. I wasn't prepared for his answer.

"I need to laugh more," he said. "I read it's better than what they'll give me. I need to stay positive."

When Dad's call came, I was living in the southwest corner of the state in Lawton, two hours away from Guthrie, and working as a reporter and wire editor at the *Lawton Constitution*. I was still in my twenties but not so young that I didn't realize what troubling ramifications Dad's news might have on our family. This wasn't just about the possibility of our family losing its patriarch but also what it could mean to lose one of my brother's main caretakers and advocates. What it could mean for Mom to be left alone with that responsibility. The immediate Hight family numbered six adult children, but we were scattered, with four still in Oklahoma but busy with our own live and families.

Dad's news was devastating to all of us, although Paul might have benefited from his belief that his prayers would heal Dad. As for me, I don't profess to know what Dad was going through. I would later learn my father was also facing the single greatest fear of a parent of an adult child with severe mental illness: *What will happen if I die?*

Four decades later, solving that problem still seems more implausible than curing cancer with laughter. Maybe, my father realized that, so he grasped onto the theory that laughter was the best medicine and didn't let go. He refused to leave his wife to deal with an adult son with mental illness. That might be too much for her. So he took the radiation treatments, the chemotherapy, and everything and anything else the doctors suggested that wouldn't make him sicker than the actual disease. He made it clear all the while that he believed a steady dose of laughter was the best protocol of the lot.

Videocassette recorders were the rave at the time, and I loaned Dad a used one I had spent a paycheck on to buy from a friend. He spent hours watching comedies, taking delight in anything funny, from the movie *Airplane* to *Caddyshack* to *9 to 5* to *Smoky and the Bandit* to *Stripes*, as well as old vaudeville classics featuring the Marx Brothers, Laurel and Hardy, and the Three Stooges. When he wasn't watching movies, the television was turned to *All in the Family*, *The Dean Martin Celebrity Roast*, *Diff'rent Strokes*, *Happy Days*, and *The Jeffersons*. When in the hospital for surgery or treatments, Dad would have the TV turned to whatever comedy he could find on the dial.

I decided to quit my job in Lawton in late 1983, a few months after the call, and temporarily move back home to be close to my parents. Home had become a stressful place, and one day to relax, I took a walk. I headed east toward a nearby Mobile gas station, not too far from where State Highway 33 intersects with Interstate 35. I walked past the garden, now much smaller and with weeds that would never have been allowed to stand when Dad had the free labor of six children. I traveled the same route my siblings and I had taken so many times to buy soft drinks, snacks, or candy in town along the same highway that Paul had tended as a flagman, the same highway that he had wandered down on so many late nights. As I neared the gas station, I saw a man with a full beard and dressed in white robes carrying a cross. I thought nothing of it—hitchhikers were, and remain, a common sight along that stretch of Interstate 35, along with individuals walking or running to raise money for a cause. Growing up, I would usually say hello to such passing strangers and continue on my way, but this man had gentle eyes and a kind face, and for some reason, I stopped.

"What are you doing in Guthrie?" I asked him.

He didn't answer me but instead said, "I see you're troubled."

"Well, a lot is going on."

"Please know you will face many obstacles and troubles in your life. Have faith. Be prayerful. God will protect you."

His eyes glowed with joy. I wondered if maybe he had a mental illness like my brother, but something about his expressions and mannerisms convinced me otherwise.

"Thank you. Who are you?"

"I am a servant of God. I'm walking to help people of faith, like you."

I thanked him for that and continued to the station, but as I walked, the man's words stayed with me, and I found myself wanting to talk with him again. I quickened my pace, rushed to make my purchase, and returned to the same spot where we had parted ways. But he was gone. For several minutes, I searched for him, but I didn't find a trace. Nonetheless, I headed home feeling uplifted and renewed.

Sources of strength, wherever they came from, were important during those days waiting to see if my father would beat cancer. Dad appeared to rely mainly on his wife and children, but he also found an interesting source of both strength and laughter in his pastor. Through the years, Dad had always had a good relationship with the parish priests who passed through Saint Mary's, but he was particularly close to Father Richard Beckman. The pastor had a dry delivery at mass and a sense a humor outside the church that Dad loved. A frequent visitor in the Hight home, Beckman once offered to give all the Saint Mary's children a ride in his shiny red convertible during a church function we hosted. When one child vomited in the car's front seat, Dad couldn't contain his laughter, one of the few times that Beckman didn't join in.

With all my father's trips to the doctor's office and the hospital, Dad and Mom hadn't been paying as much attention to other matters, and that included Paul. Stress can lead well-intentioned people to return to past coping behaviors. So maybe we shouldn't have been surprised when the voices in Paul's head started to tell him again that he didn't need his medication. He listened, and the result was predictable by now: He started to have visions. He took to wandering the streets at night. And he returned to staring at the sun.

Eventually, people noticed the change in Paul, but despite repeated pleas from family and others, Paul refused to voluntarily submit himself for treatment this time. "He was in a bad psychological state," Father Beckman said. "[Your father] wanted to care for Paul but couldn't any more. They were at odds with one another. I agreed with your father" that Paul was no longer taking his medication.

Paul became more belligerent, withdrawn, and angry—angry at his parish priest, angry at his family, angry at the world, but maybe especially angry at his father for being sick. Dad was the linchpin of the routine that had held Paul together so far, and Dad's illness had him missing in action, consumed with warding off the disease that threatened to take him away from Paul forever. Soon, we heard reports of Paul screaming at the voices again and overturning furniture in his apartment in fits of temper.

"Most everyone knew what was going on—as far as Paul's problems," Father Beckman said. "What do you do? We didn't know what to do. Most [people in the parish] didn't understand his condition. I didn't understand it either."

Despite his own serious health concerns, Dad made his focus Paul in an effort to save him. December 14, 1982, he filed a petition in Logan County District Court to force Paul back into treatment at Central State Griffin Memorial Hospital in Norman. For the first time, Dad admitted Paul's condition was worse than a chemical imbalance.

This is what he wrote in the petition filed at 3:54 p.m. that day:

> [Paul] has been treated for mental illness previously and has been diagnosed as a paranoid schizophrenic. He goes from an extreme state of depression to a very belligerent argumentative attitude. He is refusing to take his prescribed medication for his condition. He is a potential danger to himself due to a history of going into a catatonic state and lying down beside of highways.

Two days later, District Judge Bob Ward ordered the now thirty-nine-year-old Paul to be evaluated for mental illness.

Three days later, at 5:00 p.m. on December 17, Sheriff Burris delivered what was called a "notice examination and hearing" to Paul. On December 19th at 3:00 p.m., three copies of the document were delivered, one to Dad, one to Mom, and one to me. They revealed that an examining commission of two doctors had been appointed by the court to examine Paul's mental condition at a hearing scheduled for five days later at 1:00 p.m. Under Oklahoma's mental health law, the following criteria had to be established:

> a. A mentally ill person is defined as . . . any person afflicted with a substantial disorder of thought, mood perception, psychological orientation or memory that significantly impairs judgment, behavior, capacity to recognize reality, or ability to meet the ordinary demands of life.
>
> b. A person requiring treatment is defined as either: A person who has a demonstrable mental illness and who

as a result of that mental illness can be expected within the near future to intentionally or unintentionally seriously and physically injure himself or another person, or a person who has a demonstrable mental illness and who as a result of the mental illness is unable to attend to those of his basic physical needs such as food, clothing, or shelter that must be attended to in order for him to avoid serious harm in the near future and who demonstrated such inability by failing to attend to basic physical needs in the recent past.

The document stated that Paul had the right to a jury trial and a public defender if he couldn't afford an attorney. It also said Paul and the three of us could offer testimony "under oath" during the hearing. The court-appointed attorney was Brad Morelli, a family acquaintance—there were not many people in Guthrie we did not know. Years later, Morelli would recall that he ended up with many of the mental health cases because he always ate lunch at his desk, and his office wasn't far from the Logan County courthouse. Hearings for mental health cases were usually held during the noon hour and lasted forty-five minutes.

For whatever reason, my father decided to represent himself in court. Mom also decided to go, but Dad told me not to attend. I always thought he did it as a precaution, fearful that if my brother saw me in the courtroom, he might take it wrong and turn on me again.

In the meantime, Paul was taken to Central State Hospital for observation and evaluation. A doctor saw him at 10:00 p.m. Paul denied that he was having any physical problems except to say that he was allergic to his medication. But he did have an admission. "I'm hearing God's voice," Paul said. "He has a masculine, loving voice."

He then added: "I don't know why I am here."

The attendant scratched in the detention record: Paul "appears (to be) in acute distress."

Paul was put in a ward for observation, which was conducted by staff members, usually in two-hour increments. Brief notes about what they had observed included abbreviations such as "D.R." for dayroom and "wd" for ward; other symbols, such as "x" for time, were sometimes used.

Punctuation was sparse or absent in the reports, making it difficult to decipher what had been written. Still, the notes provide a glimpse into what Paul was doing at the time, with the most frequent remarks being that my brother never missed a meal or a chance for a cigarette:

Appears to be resting well.

Quiet to self. Grooming needs improving. Ate well @ noon meal.

Stays to self in day room. . . . No problems or complaints.

Quiet, up and about ward, in D.R. watching TV.

Up & about, interacts well (with) others. Showered & changed clothes.

Subject in day room at the moment smoking last cig.

About on wd, stands in one spot awhile then moves to another place. Ate breakfast.

Quiet, staying to self. Comes to aide [sic] station for smokes.

In & out of bed. Keeps to self very quietly. Is friendly when spoken to. Ate well in ward.

Pacing ward & keeping to self sits for short period of x & then paces ward.

To self in ward does appear to be in good spirits. Ate fair & (showed) unusual behavior.

Pacing hall, seems preoccupied (with) thoughts.

Up some watching TV. Keeps to self. No problems this shift.

Two days before Christmas, deputies returned Paul to Logan County District Court for his hearing. The court-appointed examining team was Dr. Jim D. Dixon and Dr. R. (Ransom) F. Ringrose. Nearing his eighty-second birthday, Dr. Ringrose was the physician who had delivered Paul and every other Hight child except for me. I was born in the hospital elevator before he arrived.

Dad was there to testify as a witness, and Paul was on the other side of the room. Mom was there too. Paul was withdrawn. In those days, Morelli met with clients in a small closet room that had two chairs amidst old files, boxes, and other junk. He said it was obvious that Paul needed serious help. Morelli asked questions such as *What's going on? Why did you get here today?* "I don't remember what he told me making a lot of sense," Morelli said. "He seemed exhausted. He was not lucid. He was in bad shape." When it was time for the hearing, the judge asked Paul whether he knew anyone in the courtroom.

"I do not know anyone!" Paul declared.

Paul had not only told Morelli his parents were dead but also that they had demons in them. Another time, Paul told the attorney that he had seen demons standing behind Mom and Dad. When the judge informed my brother that his father and mother were indeed there in the courtroom, Paul replied, "I don't have any parents or family!"

When he heard this, Dad bowed his head, and Mom's eyes turned misty. The happy child she had held in all those baby photos was now denying that she had ever existed and saying she was possessed by demons. Dad was the one who told me afterward that Paul had denied his family again. Mama wouldn't speak of it.

The doctors filed their report. Dixon wrote that Paul had begun to curse loudly more than eight weeks before. He was breaking the furniture in his apartment and seeing visions. "He is possibly dangerous to self or others as shown by past history." He recommended that Paul be hospitalized in Norman. District Judge Bob Ward concurred and ruled that the sheriff would return Paul to Norman to be committed for the second time. Morelli said that many people ended up at Norman this way, only upon their arrival to be asked one question, *Are you going to kill yourself?* If they responded, *No*, they were released immediately to return to their hometowns. Nonetheless, the judge still went through the committal process, including with Paul. "Because (he) has been committed to the state hospital by the order of the court," Ward wrote, "it is the further order of this court that his parents be allowed to enter his apartment and remove his personal effects and conclude the business of the apartment rental."

Paul would spend that Christmas, one of the holiest days in the Catholic liturgical calendar, the day Catholics gather to celebrate the birth of the Baby Jesus, alone in a room in Ward 32D of Central State Hospital. He was not allowed visitors.

* * * * *

Paul arrived at Central State Hospital alert, walking on his own, and not in acute distress, according to his records, although the report does note that "judgment and insight are poor." He was prescribed "chemotherapy (Mellaril), occupational therapy, recreational therapy, music therapy, and group therapy." He was also placed on neuroleptics, antipsychotic drugs that serve as strong tranquilizers to dull the senses and reduce confusion and agitation. Doctors also immediately placed him on a discharge plan that outlined what Paul needed to do to be released from the hospital. Paul listed his home address as my parents' and me as his only "responsible relatives."

By the end of the month, on December 30, doctors had developed a "comprehensive treatment plan" for Paul. The plan acknowledged that Paul had "problems and needs," heard the "voice of God occasionally," and had "thoughts [that] jump from one subject to another." The plan's stated goals were to prescribe chemotherapy and 150 milligrams of Mellaril with this objective:

1. Stop the voices.
2. Elevate his mood.
3. Improve his concentration through weekly

therapy sessions: three hours recreational,
three hours music, and two hours occupational.

On New Year's Eve, the state highway department removed Paul from its payroll because the formerly punctual and reliable worker had not reported to work in a month. Mom and Dad filed the forms to remove him from the state's retirement system, with one of those state forms noting, "It is our understanding that he has been committed to a mental hospital and will not return to duty."

Yet by January 3, Paul was well enough to participate in his social assessment at Central State, in which a social services worker interviewed him about his past, family, thoughts, and plans, providing some insight into what Paul was thinking at the time. The assessment revealed lapses in his thought process. Even though Paul was the oldest of seven children, he told the worker he was the oldest of five, with two brothers and two sisters. Linda was presumably missing from his list, but so was I, his youngest brother, the "responsible relative" he had named not more than a month earlier in court. He did tell the social worker all of his brothers and sisters "have done well in their own careers." He also shared that he had begun to consider the priesthood while in elementary school, had attended seminaries in San Antonio and Saint Louis, and received a *master's degree* at Saint Louis University. He mentioned his previous hospitalizations in Tulsa, Central State, and Eastern State; however, he did not mention his priesthood.

Paul did say he was now an outpatient at NorthCare Mental Health Center, and had been paying twenty dollars a month for Stelazine, an antipsychotic that treats psychotic disorders and anxiety as well as the nausea and vomiting caused by chemotherapy. He admitted he had been taking his medication until he "failed to go to get a refill." He also told the social worker about working for the state highway department and the gas station in Tulsa, which went into Phyllis Wise's report, along with how he spent his time on the outside:

In his spare time, he will read, usually magazines, or

watch some television. He has no good friends, nor does he socialize with others while he is at home. He states he is very fond of a woman friend who lives in Tulsa but feels that his illness would interfere with any plans for marriage.

The woman friend was the same Janet Lynne Brown who had cared for him when he was in Saint Francis Hospital while still in the priesthood. Paul continued to refer to her as Lynne. In one possibly surprising response, Paul said his parents were living in Guthrie and "in essentially good health." That was despite Dad still undergoing treatment for prostate cancer. "He, himself, has always been in good physical health," the social worker wrote.

The assessment's evaluation concluded: "Paul is one of a caring, concerned family. He does seem to do better when he takes his medication, but quickly has a relapse when he fails to do so. . . . He has eighteen years education but has been doing rather menial work, whereas he could probably handle a bit more challenge." Paul then revealed that he wanted to move to the Norman area and learn to play "various musical instruments." "I also want to do some work in drama, perhaps as a volunteer," he told Wise.

Wise recommended Paul as a good candidate for transitional living and vocational training. He would be referred to an outpatient mental health center in Norman. The chemotherapy and Mellaril treatments continued. But eventually the recreational, music, and occupational therapy was increased to twice a week. Paul kept insisting that he wanted to stay in Norman.

Although some of the doctors' objectives remained the same during this time, others did not. One sought to have him show "appropriate factual reflections of mood." Another sought for him to "verbalize ideas in appropriate grammatical structure (and in) accordance to sequence of events." He was reassigned to the hospital's resocialization program Monday through Friday and then put in a life adjustment course for possible job placement.

Each report said Paul had agreed with the prescribed actions. As the weeks passed, he was said to have "resolved" the voices, to have begun responding appropriately, and to be controlling his train of thought. He was still taking 150 milligrams of Mellaril. He was also asked to participate in ward and hospital activities, socialize daily, receive individual attention and counseling, and continue the life adjustment course and to seek a job in Norman. By late February 1983, one of his main activities was looking for a job. That process and continuing to take his medication continued into March.

On March 17, 1983, just two days after his father's sixty-sixth birthday, Paul completed the life adjustment course, was taking his medication regularly, and was discharged from Central State Hospital. In choppy short sentences, doctors described Paul's state of mind:

> . . . oriented to person, place, time, and situation. He is in good contact, coherent, and relevant. Speech is spontaneous and goal directed. Denies any hallucinations at this time. No loose associations of thought process and no delusional thoughts noted. Memory to recent and remote events appear intact. Insight and judgment not grossly impaired. Depression has lifted.

It was a turnaround, except again for one little note on Paul's discharge plan:

> [Paul] was unable to find work in the Norman area.

Yet again, Dad's prediction had proved true. Paul would return to Guthrie. What had not been determined was where he would live or how he would support himself without a job.

Chapter 14

The Stability Myth

On July 5, 1982, Penn Square Bank of Oklahoma City was declared insolvent, dropping what *The Oklahoman* ten years later recalled as "the biggest financial bombshell in this country since the [Great] Depression." High-living executives and risky energy loans were blamed for the closure, which devastated the banking industry and led to a lengthy congressional investigation, followed by a stream of banking reforms. Before the Eighties were over, one-fifth of all Oklahoma banks had failed, seven of Oklahoma City's ten largest banks were gone, and Oklahoma's per capita income had fallen 80 percent compared with that of the rest of the nation.

The job market collapsed in the aftermath—even for the skilled, the educated, or the connected. For a person just getting out of a mental institution, the prospects were bleak. In February 1983, Governor George Nigh issued an executive order requiring all state agencies "electing to hire, promote, or transfer employees" to justify the actions in writing, which would then be kept on file. In other words, he told them not to hire—and that included ODOT. So even with a document in hand that stated, "In the event that Mr. Hight might be able to work in the future, he will be granted reinstatement privileges if a vacant position exists," the odds of Paul being able to return to his old job weren't good. Yet in a rare lucky break, his old department came through for him.

On March 22, 1983, Paul's supervisors filed a form seeking the reinstatement of Paul *Wilbur* Hight. (Throughout their lives, Paul and our father often had *Wilber* misspelled with a "u" instead of an "e." Even family members, including me, struggled at times to spell the name correctly.)

The request stated that this "position was filled due to an immediate and necessary need for an employee to fill an approved vacancy. This employee will be used to provide maintenance for areas that will soon be under construction due to special maintenance projects. Currently their work-unit is understaffed due to frozen positions and an increased work load. This position is considered as essential and necessary to the level of service to be performed by this work-unit."

The appeal succeeded. Paul was reinstated to his former position as a transportation maintenance worker at $943 a month. He began work immediately. Looking back, the help of Paul's old boss can be seen at play. Paul told many stories about how Crabtree always urged him to take any and all training and proficiency tests that came his way. Paul took a test on fertilization and made a perfect score. He took a test on trucks and attachment certification and made a ninety-nine. Questions on that exam included how to construct a plan for snow removal, a checklist for equipment inspection, and how to back a trailer. If a written test came up, Paul was called on. Certain certifications, however, also required a physical test, something at which Paul did not excel. The trucks and attachment certification required a driving test. Paul hit five cones in three minutes thirty-three seconds. In his defense, after six months of practicing, he retook the test and didn't hit one, earning a satisfactory completion certificate. My brother had become something of an expert in this area of trucks.

His personal life, as always, was a work in progress. When Paul was first released from the hospital, he went again to live with Mom and Dad at a time when Dad was undergoing cancer treatments that left him sick at night, chilled in hot weather, and sensitive to noise. Dad grew tired of Paul's snoring, which robbed him of the little sleep he had been getting, while Mom grew weary of the rancid smell of cigarette smoke on Paul.

Little wonder that Paul began to talk about moving back into First Capitol Apartments. Dad likely would have supported the idea, but Mom would have nothing to do with it. She wanted her son living near-by so they could watch him more closely than before. She must have been determined that this time, forget all the past times, this time Paul would stay on his medications, keep his job, make some friends, and never have reason to see the inside of a courtroom again. She wanted Paul to remain at home. Dad wouldn't protest.

And there was reason for hope. Paul appeared to have benefited from the socialization training at Central State Hospital. He started to make friends beyond Lynne, who still lived more than two hours away, and began to keep in touch by letter with people he had met during his time in Norman.

In 1983, a fellow patient from Central State named John wrote to tell Paul that he was living at the downtown Oklahoma City YMCA and had found a job as a mechanic and then provided an update on his dating life. John wrote that he hadn't gone fishing yet, something Paul didn't regularly indulge in either, but he had picketed at the capitol. "That was a real joke," John wrote. "Nobody payed [sic] any attention to me. In fact, the capitol policeman said he would see me tomorrow. So much for that."

In his letter, John exhibited the qualities of a good friend, showing concern for Paul, including asking if Paul had been able to get his "old job back." John wrote he was attending Saint Joseph's Old Cathedral in downtown Oklahoma City across the street from the Oklahoma City National Memorial and Museum, the site of the April 19, 1995, bombing of the Alfred P. Murrah Federal Building:

> *I thought of you last Sunday. We had a younger priest*
> *at mass.*

John said he had joined the mailing list of the Paulist Fathers and had received a booklet from them on how to train laypeople to encourage others to join the Catholic Church. A month later, John wrote to Paul again, this time about an upcoming visit.

> *I hope to get a haircut before you come. I haven't had one since I left the hospital. Ha Ha. See you Saturday unless something comes up for you. I hope the weather is good Saturday.*
> *John*

Their correspondence appears to have ended after that or at least the letters did, but Paul was making so many new friends and rekindling so many old friendships, including ones from his past hospital stays, that our brother Bill had taken to describing Paul as a "people person." What most people looking in on his life might not have noticed, however, was that only a rare few of those people ever became close friends with Paul. Most people in his orbit were family members or priests or somehow connected to a mental health facility he had spent time in. My brother Bill recalls one fellow from a local mental health clinic who was constantly coming up with schemes for how Paul could end his days with ODOT and avoid being outside in the winter cold. "[Paul] had a peculiar way of thinking about work," Bill said. "The friend was always telling him ways not to work and get paid for it. Paul liked talking about that."

Paul, however, like so many people who work manual labor for low pay in freezing or sweltering conditions, might just have liked dreaming about going to work and sitting all day in a place where the temperature was always comfortable. A man who believed his gift was to help people, Paul might not have realized that by keeping the state's highways free of ice and in good repair, he was doing important work, keeping people safe on the road, ensuring that silly young people driving too fast in the rain made it home to their mothers. As for making more money, anyone who knew Paul knew that if he had more, he would have only given it away.

Crowded places still made Paul anxious, but he was now getting out and visiting with people, such as the waitresses at his favorite restaurant, a local cafe frequented by truck drivers who came for its simple American staples: pancakes, chicken-fried steak, burgers. Bill ate there with Paul more than once and found the experience to be revealing. "This food is terrible," Paul whispered to Bill. "The service is terrible too." The Hight children had been taught never to complain about food out loud and to eat everything on their plates as quickly as possible. Paul always excelled at the later, devouring whatever was served to him, even when not particularly appetizing. On this day, despite his comments about the food, Paul insisted on paying the bill and left a big tip for the waitress. A puzzled Bill raised an eyebrow and said with a slight frown, "Why did you do that? You said the food was terrible."

Technically, Paul had said the *service* was terrible too, but he just replied, "They don't make any money here, and I like this place!" Paul then took one more bite of the few remaining morsels on his plate and said with an onerous smirk, "This food is *really* terrible."

The thing was, said Bill, the next time he visited Guthrie, Paul wanted to go to the same place. The old Cheers theme song used to sing about the joy of going someplace where everybody knows your name. Maybe that Guthrie café was Paul's Cheers, a café, not a bar, but nonetheless, a place where people were happy to see him and to chat, a place where he felt welcome—where his mental illness didn't matter.

* * * * *

In August 1985, Paul decided he needed a new, more economical car, mainly for getting to work or making the long drive to visit Lynne. The '75 Impala was getting cranky and using too much gasoline. The only problem was this meant buying a car. Now that was something our father loved to do. For years, the Hights had bought their cars at Austin Chevrolet in downtown Guthrie, where Dad was known for kicking the tires and wheeling and dealing on the price. But Paul balked at the tradition and instead went on his own to Country Chrysler in Guthrie. He found a Dodge Aries and bought it. He wasn't mechanical, so he didn't look at the engine or kick the tires. He didn't care much about money, so he didn't wheel or deal. He didn't question the price tag of the car or check the Blue Book price because he trusted just about everyone, especially a salesman with the name of the brother who visited him so often. Salesman Bill sold the car to Paul for $9,850.

Unbeknownst to just about everyone, including the family, Paul had started to save money, enough by living at home to make a hefty down payment on the car. He wrote a check for $4,000 and then received $800 for his old Impala. After agreeing to buy fabric protection because he often dropped his cigarettes and coffee on the seats, Paul financed the car for $5,200. Buying that car and doing it his way and not his father's were signs that Paul was becoming more self-sufficient and, in a little way, more his own man. Being able to buy that car on his own was proof that if Paul took his medication, he could be independent, make friends, and hold a steady job, even if the latter wasn't exactly what he wanted in a job.

Yes, 1985 was turning out to be a good year for the Hights. Paul was stable and driving a new car, and not long after that, Dad announced that his laughter therapy had worked: His cancer was in remission. He and Mom had endured three years of hell battling the insidious disease on top of fifteen years dealing with the fallout of Paul's illness. They agreed it was time to retire. Dad was sixty-eight years old. Mom, sixty-five. Both were still relatively young and able to travel.

Dad said he wanted to buy an RV or a fifth-wheel travel trailer that he could attach to the back of a pickup so they could go to bluegrass festivals and on excursions with friends. Mom was not against the idea but also looked forward to puttering around her flower beds and the acreage; she was also still holding out for that dream trip to Hawaii. Although journalism is rarely a path to great riches, I continued to hold to my promise that if Dad didn't do it first, I would someday take her to the Aloha State. The rest of their lives awaited—a well-earned period of leisure and travel and time spent with their children and grandchildren. Their daughters had already given them four grandchildren, and Dad held out hope that one of his sons would provide a grandchild to carry on the Hight name. He had started asking me when I was going to find someone to marry. Mom, as always, said she wanted me to be happy and more stable myself.

Stability had been an elusive Holy Grail for the Hight family, including for me. My five years in journalism had been anything but stable. I had quit a job in protest, seen a weekly newspaper shut down by ownership, and been fired from another for a well intentioned, satirical column. I had achieved the trifecta of a journalistic career at age twenty-six. Yet 1985 brought an upswing in stability for me as well. After I had freelanced for several months at the state's largest newspaper, *The Oklahoman*, hired me full time as a metro reporter. I moved out of my parents' house and into an apartment with a college friend in Oklahoma City.

In 1985, for the first time in many years, Christmas was a happy one for the entire Hight family, especially Mom. Paul was still smoking, to her displeasure, but he was once again jovial and joking as we gathered before the tree, and that meant her oldest son was relatively stable, which is all Mom asked. It was an unexpected blessing that her newest granddaughter, Rebecca, was celebrating her first Christmas with them too.

Mom spent much of the day playing with the baby, who looked so much like Linda at that age, the joy had to be bittersweet. Only a parent who had lost a child could know what Mom was thinking as the two of them cooed and played.

Late that afternoon as I went to leave, Mom seemed deservedly tired from the day's festivities. A house full of Hights is a wonderful thing but also a good deal of work. Yet Mom looked radiant as I waved good-bye and promised to see her in a couple of days. "I love you, Mama," I said, pausing at the door to look back one last time.

For so many years, those three words had remained understood between us but never said, until seven months before, when at the end of a phone call, I decided to say, "I . . . love . . . you, Mama." A moment passed before she replied, "Well, we love you too." We had been saying those words ever since, and our relationship had deepened, possibly as a result. We were closer and more frank with each other now. We talked about finances, relationships, religion, family, and even Paul's ever-changing ups and downs, which my parents for so long had tried to protect me from. In one of our calls, Mom made a point to say she would be there for me, including the day I married. She had become my best friend.

On my twenty-seventh birthday, my mother gave me a card that read on the front, "For a wonderful son on his birthday." Inside were these words: "Family life is many things, and one of the nicest joys it brings is having a son as wonderful as you, who's thought of in a special way, not only on a special day, but warmly and with love the whole year through!" She wrote in her familiar handwriting at the end, "We love you—Daddy & Mama."

That Christmas afternoon, as my three little words reached her, Mom looked up at me with her soft blue eyes and smiled. The natural beauty Dad had spotted more than forty years ago at Saint Mary's could still be seen. "Merry Christmas, Joe," she said. And as she had said on that first call seven months earlier and so many times since, "I love you too!"

Mom had had the truly merry Christmas she deserved. I was stable after five tumultuous years. Paul's condition was stable. Our family was stable. God was smiling upon our family again.

Not a day later, I would drive back to Guthrie in a haze. I had received another phone call from my father, only this one was an early morning call at my work. His trembling voice was much more urgent this time. The call wasn't about him. It wasn't about Paul. He told me I needed to come home immediately.

"Why?"

"Your mother died in her sleep."

I would never fully trust stability again.

Chapter 15

Heartbreak and New Beginnings

Mom had never liked going to doctors. They were expensive and usually only gave bad news. She had gotten so much bad news through the years, she probably couldn't bear to hear any more. She was also a typical mother: she always put everyone else's needs before her own.

And, of course, there were the losses, oh, so many losses.

The toll the death of a child takes on a parent might have been known anecdotally when Linda died all those years ago, but such tragedies certainly weren't readily talked about, studied, or understood in the 1940s. No parish grief group existed to provide support. No national online Compassionate Friends group connected grieving parents with other grieving parents. No grief expert, almost no books, stood ready to explain how the loss of a child could haunt your nights and reappear each new day, every day . . . until the end of your days.

My mother had to find her own way out of grief, with only the help of her grieving husband and her family and her faith. When mental illness took hold of her oldest son and took away her son as she had known him, that was a different kind of loss. With mental illness, the son she knew would reappear every so often, only to have the illness snatch him away again. Each disappearance was a little death, packaged with a never-ending litany of trouble and woe until one day that beloved firstborn was standing before the world denying her as his mother.

By the early hours of December 26, 1985, the heartbreaks of life had weakened my mother's heart to the point that it was barely beating. Dad said that in recent days, Mom had mentioned feeling more tired than ever, with some pain in her chest and arms. I had noticed a weariness about her that Christmas afternoon as I left her. But Mom never said a word, never complained to anyone but Dad. In truth, such pains were nothing for a woman who had suffered the losses she had.

On Christmas night, she knelt by her bed as she had done so many times. She probably thanked God for the joy of that Christmas Day. She probably thanked God for healing her husband and his continued good health. She probably mentioned each child and grandchild by name and asked God to protect each one. She would not have prayed for herself, except to ask that she be allowed to join Linda, her parents, and the rest of her family in heaven someday. On slipping into bed, she whispered to Dad that she loved him before drifting off and into the most peaceful, everlasting sleep of her life.

For my father, finding his beloved wife dead in their marital bed was a wall he couldn't see past. He could only see the past. The daughter who had tragically died. The son whose mind had been tragically altered. And now the wife who, as the Bible described, had been taken by death like a thief in the night. He might have also blamed, if only for a moment, the weight of the trials of his oldest son for hastening his wife's death, as he had blamed that son so many years ago for taking Linda to the water tank. What is known for sure is that Dad remained strident in his Catholic faith, and as he had done when his little daughter died, he turned to the Bible for answers.

He read this verse from Corinthians:

For this momentary affliction is preparing for us an eternal weight of glory beyond all comparison, because we look not to the things that are seen but to the things

160

that are unseen; for the things that are seen are transient, but the things that are unseen are eternal.

Yet in the end, it was Corinthians where he found what he must do:

Be watchful, stand firm in your faith, be courageous, be strong.

Dad resolved to stand resolute, for himself and his family. Such resolve was not so easy for his youngest son to find. I was left stunned, shell-shocked. How could my mother, who had looked so radiant just the day before, be dead? As I drove home, I screamed at God for answers. I was only twenty-seven years old. I was supposed to take Mom to Hawaii. I was supposed to have her in the front pew when I wed. I was supposed to have a grandma for my children as my sisters had. Now that wasn't going to happen, couldn't happen. Through my tears, I asked for answers too. But unlike those who hear voices, none came for me.

Indeed, the only one of the family who seemed accepting of Mom's death was Paul, who moved through the days that followed as if he knew something the rest of us didn't. "Mom is in heaven," he said.

Did my brother know this because the voices had told him or was he calling on the words he had used as a priest to comfort those who had suffered a loss? In the end, where his faith came from probably didn't matter. What was surprising was that Paul, the one had been rejected by the Church, seemed the only Hight steadfast in the belief that God had taken Mom to be with him and Linda. Once again, my father planned a funeral—an echo in many ways of the first. The rosary was held on the evening of December 27, Paul's birthday, at Davis Funeral Home, a new name but where Linda had also lain. The Funeral Mass was at Saint Mary's.

Still in a haze, I floundered, trying to find solace in something. Mom had always dreaded growing older and becoming a burden on her children. She feared drifting into Alzheimer's as her own mother had. At sixty-five, though, she had still been young, too young—her family still needed her. I know I did. "It was her time, Joe. She died in peace. She's in heaven now," Paul said. I believed my brother, I did. Yet I struggled to accept her unexpected death.

After the rosary, we gathered around Mom's casket to say our final good-byes. Paul was right; she did look peaceful. That did not, however, stay the tears for me or for my brothers and sisters—not even Paul. The room emptied, but we couldn't bring ourselves to leave the funeral home. The next day, the casket would be closed. We would not see our mother on this earth again.

"We have to go," Dad finally said. "We have to move on from this."

We followed him down the aisle and out of the chapel. I glanced back one last time, remembering the smile Mom and I had exchanged on Christmas Day. "I love you," I said.

The next morning, on a mild winter's day, Dad led us down the long aisle of Saint Mary's to the front of the church. I stared at the floor, unable to look at anyone. We were all in pain, but no one can know another's grief or how it manifests itself in anyone but you. I couldn't imagine what our father was going through. This was the church where he had been smitten by a young Pauline Kingston, the same church where he had buried his oldest daughter and had celebrated his oldest son becoming a priest. Briefly, I wondered how Paul, the priest, would have handled such a Mass for his own mother.

We buried Mom next to Linda at Summit View Cemetery, near the graves of Mom's parents. Dad's spot beside Mom waited for him. What went unsaid was the fear that the stress of losing Mom, combined with his own health issues, might cause that day to come sooner. Still, Paul remained matter-of-fact, if finally emotional. At one point, Jerry Lindsley, his friend, suggested, "Let's go out to the cemetery to see your mother."

"No!" Paul shouted. "She's not there anyway." But if someone had asked, he would have said she was in heaven.

Sooner than we were probably ready, everybody returned to work and our individual lives. My strength in the days that followed came through the young adult group I had joined through the archdiocese and Edmond's Saint John the Baptist Catholic Church. Calling my father and siblings triggered too many emotions. Occasionally, Paul would call to see how I was doing. "It's pretty rough here. Daddy's having a hard time," he would say, "but Mama's looking down on all of us. She's smiling because she's in heaven with Linda. I know that."

His words rang hollow for me. I found it difficult to believe the shadow of Mom's death would ever lift. Then a little more than a month later, in early February, I started to notice a young woman with a radiant smile at Saint John's. At first, we talked only briefly, mostly at the young adult group, but that soon grew into longer conversations. She soon asked me to go to the Sadie Hawkins dance. Two weeks later, I asked her to marry me. I had yet to meet her parents. At the time, some people questioned whether we were rushing into marriage, whether I was rushing into it because of my mother's recent death. Their concerns didn't worry me; I knew Nan Bloch was perfect for me, even though we were different in many ways. I was from a big family in a small town. She was from a small family in Oklahoma City. She often repeated the words of her mother, "City-born and city-bred, and when I die, I'll be city-dead."

I was a journalist. She was a musician and a school band director. In other words, we would never have a lot of money. At the time, I was making $21,000 a year and hadn't saved a dime in my life. My first visit to meet her parents, Henry and Mary Louise Bloch, made it clear to me that this country boy would be marrying into a family that knew how to set the table properly (and did so at every meal) and how to dress and act on formal occasions. Yet because their daughter had declared her love for me, they accepted me immediately. The Blochs were what rural folks in Oklahoma call good people.

Before our wedding, Nan and I took the Pre-Cana course required by the Catholic Church. We answered many questions in writing, including some pointed ones. I wrote that I admired Nan's kindness and caring attitude, her love and commitment to God, and her ability to laugh, which often seemed triggered by my awkwardness around her parents.

Our wedding was scheduled in September. On my side of the family, Paul was jubilant and readily accepted Nan. Bill and John did too, and Dad did as well, mainly because our relationship recalled his own courtship with Mom. My sisters, however, were more reserved. Years later, however, Marilyn would loudly proclaim, "That Nan has sure classed Joe up."

While we prepared for the wedding, my brother Paul was experiencing the despair of a suicide epidemic in Oklahoma. The shenanigans that had taken down Penn Square Bank, created a state bank crisis, and roiled the national economy had also led to a farm crisis in Oklahoma by the mid-1980s. With farmers' great reliance on debt to finance farm operations, the fates of banks and family farms were critically intertwined. How could the outcome be any other way? Soon the state was losing more than four family farms a day. Corporate and personal bankruptcies skyrocketed. Suicides in Oklahoma topped the national average, and they were twice as high for farmers.

The stories, which blazed across front pages of the state's newspapers, were horrific: The forty-year-old son of a prominent banker who had lost all of his family's land killed himself, his wife, and ten-year-old child. Police found his diary with the word *responsible* written on the last page. A fifty-four-year-old kindergarten teacher with a farm facing foreclosure was found dead, her body strewn across a burning trash heap. A fifty-year-old banker killed himself in his bank's offices.

Those suicides were mental suffering for all the world to see. Meanwhile, Paul, in his trips to Central State and mental health clinics across Oklahoma, was trying to help others, to fight the stage of the illness before the suicide, like a doctor trying to heal cancer before it goes to the lymph nodes and can't be stopped. He talked to people to counsel them as he would have when he was a priest. The task must have felt overwhelming. Paul spoke of an executive vice president of a rural Oklahoma bank who killed himself, after which the man's oldest son did the same.

What effect all this unnecessary loss had on Paul, I cannot say, but I do know he did what he could to help, and he kept up a good front. Maybe in the face of such a statewide tragedy that touched the lives of rural people so like the ones he had grown up with, being able to console the victims helped him keep his own mental health issues at bay during this time. According to the National Alliance on Mental Health, studies have shown that helping others can help ease depression. I only know my brother was cheerful when I asked him if he could do the two readings at my wedding. His booming, distinct voice at the ceremony would remind me of the big brother from my childhood. I also asked my brother Bill to read a poem I had written to Nan the week before our wedding.

On September 20, 1986, at Saint John's, we wed. I thought of my mother as I sat in the sanctuary. Nan looked as radiant as she walked down the aisle as she had the first time I looked into her eyes. The wedding was flawless, until Nan slid my wedding band onto the wrong finger. We both laughed. Those in the pews roared. Then all fell silent again as Paul read the scripture, Father Joe Ross gave his homily about the joining of a couple as one, and Bill began to read the poem I had dedicated to Nan:

> They are strangers
> Born in different places and times.
> For many years, the strangers' walks of life never cross.
> They are loved
> And cared for by others.
> They live in a world without the other.
> For it is not the time nor the place for them to meet.
>
> Sometimes at night
> Tears trickle down the strangers' faces, and they
> wonder about their lives.
> The dream of the perfect love, but it's not there.
> They feel their struggles are many,
> And their victories are few.
> And, finally, they bend their knees and look up to the sky.
> Who am I, Lord? they ask,
> Where is my love upon this earth?

A compassionate God looks upon the strangers,
And touches them.
Don't worry, He says. Soon, that love will be there.

One day, the strangers' paths cross.
They glance into each other's eyes.
Their voices speak a timid *hello*.
And their smiles tingle in anticipation
 of meeting someone new.
The strangers begin to talk,
And they enjoy short moments together.
They begin discovering the depths of each other's hearts.
They find similar struggles.
And they cry together,
In sadness and in joy.

As the days and months pass,
the strangers begin looking for each other in crowds.
Their eyes sparkle when they're together.
They find beauty in each other
That no one else had seen before.
The strangers know
There's much more to discover about the other.
But they look into each other's eyes
And promise to love forever.

Down an aisle they walk,
And they kneel together.
They look up to the sky,
I am here, Lord, they say. I have found my love.
And God looks down on the two, and says,
Strangers they are no more.
They are friends.
And today I join them together, as one.

As Bill finished the poem, I heard my father choking up behind me as well as sniffles in the crowd. A breeze brushed the back of my neck. Only a breeze? Or my mother's spirit fulfilling the promise she had made to me only months before that she would be there on my wedding day?

I felt the breeze once more, as if my mother were reaching out to me. As if she were there with me. As if she were saying to me one more time, "I love you too, Joe."

Chapter 16

No Longer Our Home

Nan and I drove to the house that was no longer my home for the auction in 1988. My mother had been dead for less than three years. The house and surrounding five acres, next to the adjoining property owned by her parents in east Guthrie, had been her domain. She had lived on it most of her married life and had turned it into a haven for stray cats and dogs, opossums and birds, and her own adult children as needed. As we drove up, a hummingbird flitted about one of the many bird feeders she and my father had put up over the decades.

The place teemed with memories: Mom and I watching a funnel cloud swirl above our heads before it drifted away. Mom by a small pen, without hesitation grabbing the tail of a skunk threatening our puppies and whirling the stinky intruder into the yard. Mom in my room, scolding me for the perpetual mess. Mom consoling me after I buried the tiny puppy born with a birth defect.

This was the land where my mother had thrived and land that she had protected with her very being. Now Dad was ready to sell it and everything on it. I considered buying the property, if only because of how deeply my mother cared about it. The acreage was worth the $60,000

Dad wanted for it. However, buying the old family spread would have meant a much longer drive to work, along with Nan's uneasiness about living in a rural setting. To be candid, I wasn't sure I relished the notion of returning to Guthrie either.

Dad's idea to sell the house took time to become a reality. Despite his desire to move forward after Mom's death—if only for the sake of his family, Dad did not immediately do so. He holed up at home at first, with Paul as his only companion and the occasional visits of friends, such as Father Beckman. My brother Bill came home one day to find Dad on the couch alone, watching a football game on TV. He barely recognized this quiet, homebound man as the father who was always meeting and greeting people and bull-shooting.

"You need to get out more," Bill told him.

"Yes, I do," Dad said, adding. "I want to travel."

That encounter with Bill seemed to unlock a door. A few days later, Dad bought an old Suburban and a fifth-wheel Nomad trailer. He began to go fishing with friends and Bill. Family photographs capture father and son wearing matching Padre Island ball caps, holding a long line of fish that they had caught near the island. The fishing trips were only the beginning. Dad started to attend bluegrass concerts and then dances and other social events. He took to leading weekly Bible studies at the house. And at the age of seventy-one, Dad began to date. He still at times mentioned a desire to travel the country but had yet to venture too far from home.

Paul, still living at home, became the pipeline to the latest news about Dad's antics. Paul would call to report: Did you know Dad did this? And did I tell you Dad went there? For his siblings, Paul was like having a personal reporter on site. It wasn't too long until an unexpected report came in: Dad was seeing a new woman, one he seemed particularly interested in. Joy Streck Anderson lived in a three-bedroom house across the street from her mother in Hennessey, a farming community about forty-five miles northwest of Guthrie. She had moved to town from a farm after losing her husband. She worked in the oil fields, which were popping up in the area, checking wells for a Hennessey woman, and she would be the first to say that she was settled in her life until one of her uncles came to her in 1987 with a suggestion.

"I've met this nice man you should meet," he said.

"I don't want no man," said Joy, whose Oklahoma accent was more distinctly rural and southern than ours. "I don't plan to date or marry again."

"Well, he's really nice. Let me check him out, and I'll let you know."

Joy, who could be timid like our mother at times, reluctantly let her uncle talk her into it. A few days later, the uncle returned with a report: "I've talked to a lot of people who all say Wilber Hight is the nicest man they've ever met." Joy agreed to have supper, as she called it, with Dad, and shortly thereafter, they had a date at a diner in Enid, the area's largest city at more than 45,000 people.

Dad said he was immediately impressed by Joy, if only because she liked the diner's giant hamburgers. If at first glance the fifty-six-year-old, five-foot-eight-inch, big-boned Joy seemed the exact opposite of my petite mother, upon a closer look, it was clear they shared the important qualities. Like Mom, Joy had a caring, hardworking nature and a quick laugh when it came to Dad's storytelling and jokes.

Soon Dad was spending all his time with Joy, even accompanying her to the oil wells. Although not born a Catholic, Joy became interested in becoming one. In the official eyes of the Catholic Church, that would have been a requisite for marriage. Whether Dad saw it that way is another story.

And then one evening while checking the wells together, a gas line ruptured, sending the pipe waving in the air. For Joy, the rupture was no big deal. For Dad, such dangers shouldn't be part of any job. He took one look at the line whistling in the Oklahoma wind, looked at Joy, and declared, "Quit these damn oil wells, marry me, and let's travel!"

They were married on Saturday, November 7, 1987, at Saint Mary's, where Dad had married Mom, baptized his children, buried his daughter, attended Paul's ordination and first Mass and his children's weddings, and married Mom. Paul was Dad's best man. Saint Mary's new pastor, Father Elmer Carl Robnett, who had served as a paratrooper during World War II and been personally responsible for bringing some six thousand Vietnamese refugees to Oklahoma, starting in 1975, celebrated the Mass.

With some twenty immediate family members looking on, Father Robnett read from the "Together for Life" booklet that included the Catholic rite of marriage, which had been revised in 1969 as part of the post–Vatican II changes. Paul, wearing a tan dress coat and brown tie, held the same booklet throughout the ceremony. With head bowed, eyes closed, Paul prayed when Robnett prayed. He read silently when Robnett read. If my brother had still been a priest, he would have performed the ceremony himself, and so the day was once again, whether the words were spoken or not, set against a backdrop of loss—of a wife and mother, a priesthood, and a child—as all Hight occasions had been for so long and would forever be. Yet the relief of Paul's mental illness being in check during this critical time for our father was a blessing all its own.

After the wedding, Dad and Joy went to stay at my Aunt Elvrie's home in California. One morning at about four o'clock, an earthquake rattled their bed and awakened Dad.

"Get ready," he told Joy, "we're going home!"

And that they did, not stopping until they were safely back in Oklahoma with another story to add to his repertoire.

* * * * *

Dad had fallen in love and remarried faster than many in the family would have expected, having buried the love of his life less than two years earlier. Yet he did not hesitate to ask all of us children to accept Joy immediately as the new matriarch of our family. Dad's request was difficult for most of us, as we were still grieving the loss of our mother, but somehow not for Paul, even though Joy had been forewarned that he "might throw a ring-tailed fit" about the marriage. Paul was still living at home when Joy arrived to settle into the east Guthrie house. Dad hadn't provided much warning, and Joy didn't know much about Paul's condition.

Still, today, she says with emphasis in her voice, "Paul became my buddy. I had no fear of him." As for Paul, he began to call her Mom immediately, while the rest of my siblings and I continued to use her first name. Every day, Paul would return home from his work for ODOT asking, "Mom, what's for dinner?"

Harmony continued until one day, while Paul was in the kitchen with them, Dad snuck a kiss from Joy. Paul's face reddened at the display of affection, followed by a look of outrage. He stormed outside without saying a word. A few nights later, Joy looked up from their bed to see Paul's shadow in the doorway, reminiscent of the visits he used to make to my room when I was a child, and the reason I still always shut and locked my door at night. When Joy told Dad about the latest incident, my father exclaimed, "You lock the door from now on when you're in there!"

Not long afterward, Dad decided he needed to get away from Paul, the old family home, and Guthrie. The old Suburban and Nomad trailer were his answer. Dad signed up for the Good Sam's Club, basically a community for the RV crowd, and quickly became nearly as staunch a "Good Sam" as he was a Catholic. By then, Dad and Joy were traveling the country and into Canada with five or six other couples, and before long, Dad returned home wearing the floppy hat signifying that he had been elected president of the local club. Those excursions were made possible by old trusted friends back home who Dad knew would call him if something were ever to happen to Paul.

All, however, was not unanimous on the home front. Joy thought the Nomad was too small for a home, and Dad thought living at the Guthrie house was too much. The house still reminded him of Mom, and he was also worried that his oldest son who lived there was becoming too attached to his new wife. Dad decided he could no longer live in the east Guthrie house, nor could he subject Joy to living in the same home and bedroom that had been Mom's domain. He decided to move to Hennessey, with its one grocery store, its farming and oil culture, and its community where everyone knew his new wife. He would live in Joy's home. He summoned his children to a drawing for furniture, including the pieces he had built himself, and other family possessions—everyone except Paul. Dad continued to maintain that Paul would either fail to care for any treasure received or would give it away. Everyone else would end up with two items, and the rest would be sold at auction, where we were free to bid on items with the rest of Guthrie.

That decision rocked the stability of the Hight family again—and not only for Paul, who would soon not have a place to live. The day of the auction found our childhood placed out for sale on the lawn. Everything familiar to us was for sale: the old red Ford tractor Dad had sat on for so many hours tending his garden. The rocker that he favored during the evening and early morning hours when he was lecturing us, watching TV, or couldn't sleep. The antique Wells Fargo safe where Mom had stored the family's paperwork and some of her safety money. As Nan and I approached the sale, a few hours before the auction began, I could see most of the rest of the family had also arrived. My brothers and sisters gathered in the living room for one last time. Everyone was tense. When Dad walked in, almost everyone started yelling at him. Some questioned the injustice of him doing this to his children. Some were offended by the dismantling of Mom's home. Some wondered why Dad was okay with erasing their past, their family's past—in essence, the history of the Pauline and Wilber Hight family.

Dad's reply echoed what he had said at Mom's funeral: "I just can't live here anymore. I have to leave this house, this town, this place. I loved your mother, but I have to move on."

The yelling continued—and I don't remember anyone asking about Paul or what he thought or where he would go once the house was gone; I don't remember Paul participating at all. Maybe he stepped outside or faded into the background, unwilling to engage.

"Stop!" I finally yelled. "He has every right to sell this place! We may not like it, but he has the right!"

I stormed out. Everyone else did too. I would not return to that living room until years later, and then only as an invited guest.

When the bidding began, Nan and I were there to see it, and we watched almost until the end. We put in a few unsuccessful bids. Dad's best-seat-in-the-house rocking chair was my lone prize of the daylong auction. My brothers and sisters won other items, but I don't think Paul bid on a thing. He just watched from afar with a cigarette in his mouth, I would learn later that he was thinking about how he had helped Dad build the house. Our family left the auction without saying another word to each other. It felt like Mom's funeral all over again—only this time, Paul was left without a home.

By September 1988, my oldest brother had moved back into First Capitol Apartments in Guthrie, only this time in unit No. 11, next door to the one he had trashed during his psychotic episode five years before. Despite all the family upheaval and the disruption to his routine, he remained stable. He still worked at ODOT. He was, however, now in his late forties, and the injuries from hard outside work had begun to accumulate: A finger lacerated on a truck's closing tailgate. A back injury brought on from lifting a heavy water can. Another back injury.

The injuries and treatment caused Paul to miss work, but despite this, Paul continued to receive glowing evaluations from Crabtree, including an entry noting that Paul had scored the highest in the department's division on an herbicide test. "He strives to be helpful to the moving crew by assisting repairs to mowing equipment, acting as a flag person, and putting up signs for safety control. His easygoing manners and attitude make him a pleasure to the entire crew and supervisor," Crabtree wrote. "Paul continues to strive to develope [sic] improvement in all job tasks he undertakes. He is an inspiration to our crew and to all who come in contact with him."

Paul penned a grateful response to his boss as he had before, writing that Crabtree was "a great supervisor," and he was working with "a great crew." And aside from the physical injuries incurred at work, Paul was doing well during this period.

In early 1989, our father got one of his big ideas, this one involving the old family acreage and Paul. Although the three acres where the east Guthrie house stood had been sold, the adjoining two acres, where Mom's parents had lived, remained in the family. The old house had been demolished, the land cleared, and a foundation poured for a trailer house. A couple had moved in, and Dad asked the tenants if they would be interested in selling it. They were. Only eight months after Paul had returned to First Capitol Apartments, he moved again, only this time into his own home. Paul's first home purchases were a brown La-Z-Boy and a big-screen TV. Whether Paul purchased the trailer home or Dad did with the intention of renting it to Paul is unknown; no paperwork was ever filed on the home or property. Ironically, my brother Bill contends Paul never wanted the mobile home, that the first home of his own was forced on our brother.

"I don't like it," Paul told Bill. "I don't want to stay here."

In the end, Paul's wishes went unheard. Dad's will being the stronger of the two, Paul was soon back living on the family land as Dad wanted. He tried to find his way back to stable again, despite being all on his own. Thankfully, Paul continued to take his medication during this time, and his life followed a routine not unlike many in the country's heartland. When not watching TV, he was either reading the Bible or taking notes about what he was watching on TV, usually various televangelists, usually with a cup of coffee nearby. He also took time to make notes about his thoughts and other musings. He jotted all this in notebooks, on notepads or any scrap of available paper. Some notes were reminders of future important dates; some, of the past. On an Oklahoma Highway Credit Union notepad, he wrote:

Best friend Stephanie. Anniversary date, June 20, 1990, at Saint Mary's Church in Guthrie. 3:30 p.m. Paul W. Hight.

No one ever figured out who this best friend was or if she existed.

During this time, Paul took to sitting outside on the porch and having a smoke. He was smoking Marlboros now; with a nearly $1,100 monthly income, he could afford them. He developed a habit of walking to the nearby gas station for cigarettes, Pepsi, or a snack. His home—and everything in it—still reeked of cigarette smoke, but he made a point of not smoking when he had guests over or when he was a guest in someone else's home, leftover habits from living at his parents' house where smoking had been prohibited.

Paul never had a lot of habits, good or bad, nor did he have many hobbies. He did, however, enjoy debating Scripture with any Jehovah's Witnesses, Mormons, or any other denomination representatives who happened to knock on his door. That was a more frequent occurrence than you might think, given that Paul lived right off the highway. Unlike most people, who might try to pretend they weren't home or tell them to go away, Paul welcomed the missionaries into his home.

"He would quote Scripture to them and back them down," Bill said, although he couldn't expound on what points Paul was trying to make with his visitors. Still, no one disputed our brother's knowledge of Scripture, something for which, unlike their Protestant peers, lay Catholics are not known. That included our father, who had also suddenly rediscovered a heightened interest in reading the Holy Book.

Because of the cigarette stench, Bill was the only family member who would stay at Paul's. He made the two-hour drive from Bartlesville regularly for holidays and visits as long as Paul remained there. On those visits, Bill recalled that Paul would always want to go out, to a restaurant, a movie, an exhibit, even the pet store—things Paul rarely did by himself.

Otherwise, Paul was mostly on his own.

And without his mother watching over him and making sure he took his medicine and with Dad away in Hennessey, Paul started to revert to his old ways. He went off his medication and soon became belligerent. He took to wandering the highways at night again. And then his friend Jerry Lindsley heard that Paul had allowed a stranger, a man found wandering the highway, to stay two or three days with him in his home. That hospitality might have been a part of Paul's new routine, but the end result wasn't a good one for him or for anyone else.

Dad received one of those phone calls he dreaded.

We all dreaded them.

He and Joy set out for Guthrie uncertain of what they would find.

Chapter 17

The Mysterious Diagnosis

The drive from Hennessey to Guthrie recalls the barren Texas roads that Tom Hanks travels in the final scenes of the movie *Cast Away*. As Hanks's character Chuck Noland is told, you'll see a whole lot of nothing. Although maybe it's more accurate to say nothing worth remembering: oil derricks, oil tankers, endless wheat fields, the occasional farmhouse or trailer, a rare tree or thicket—the kind of monotonous scenery that can lull a driver to sleep but one that also possesses the lonely beauty of an Andrew Wyeth painting.

For Joy and Dad, the trip to Paul's took about forty-five minutes, but it surely felt more like hours. Dad had expressed a desire to avoid these repetitive and tedious trips to see or rescue his oldest son. He wanted to be on the open road headed elsewhere, far away from his past life, far away from Paul's endless troubles.

When Dad was not traveling with Joy and their new friends, he settled into a more rural life than he had previously known in Guthrie. Soon, like his new wife, everyone in Hennessey knew him. A regular at Sunday Mass at Saint Joseph Catholic Church, Dad became a leader in the parish but not so much that it might interfere with his latest travel plans. Parked outside their brown brick home in Hennessey was now a new red GMC pickup truck and a longer fifth-wheel with an expanded living area. Dad had bought it with proceeds from the auction of the east Guthrie home that he had built with his own hands, and the help of Paul. Using any reasonable standard, Dad's life was good again, with one exception: the continued irritation of Paul and his troubles.

According to the phone call that had precipitated this trip to his son's, Paul had been off his medication for about eight days. In a new twist, Paul had taken to dropping lighted cigarettes on himself, in his car, and in his home—a fire seemed inevitable. My brother was also hearing voices again, and from what Logan County Sheriff Burris had said in his call to Dad, the voices weren't particularly thrilled with life in Guthrie and had been pestering Paul to let everyone know about their displeasure. Unsatisfied with Paul's progress on the matter, the voices had demanded that Paul prove to everyone in a dramatic manner that he was not happy, hence the tiny fires. Dad told the sheriff to take Paul into custody and then to the crisis center. Paul was facing another court-ordered detention in a mental institution.

When Dad and Joy finally arrived at Paul's that day, they found he had fulfilled the latest command of the voices. He had tossed his furniture and big-screen TV into a nearby creek. The front door of his house was open, and the contents that remained inside were either overturned or had been thrown against the wall. Only Paul's Bible and some notes beside it on a small side table were undisturbed. Burglars could not have ransacked a home any better. Dad's travels would be restricted to Paul's house and court for the near future.

A hearing to order Paul back to Griffin Memorial Central State Hospital was scheduled for June 2, 1989, and that request was approved. For the first time in six years, Paul was headed back to Norman. The setback was painful—Paul had managed to survive Mom's untimely death and absence, buoyed by his belief in God and his conviction that Mom was safe and happy in heaven with Linda. But Dad's decision to sell the family home, move away from Guthrie, and move Paul into a home he didn't want, far away from everyone else in the family, might have been too much for Paul to handle. A judge ruled that Paul was a danger to himself and not competent to submit to voluntary treatment. He was ordered for treatment not to exceed twenty-eight days.

At Central State, doctors again evaluated Paul and his mental state. He had been going to the Wheatland Mental Health Center in Guthrie regularly twice a month and had continued to take the 150 milligrams of Mellaril that had kept him stable for the last six years. However, without the medication, in a matter of eight days, Paul was back to hearing voices—voices that bombarded him with threats such as "someone was going to kill him" and "aliens from other planets will take over the U.S." As the report said, "It seems that the voices that talk to him are similar to the people that he knows, and he becomes more suspicious."

Paul was placed in a ward for observation and was questioned more. He denied not having an appetite, which was probably true, given his natural voracious one. He also denied he was suffering from insomnia. Denied being depressed. Denied being suicidal . . . denied being continuously suicidal. Despite the latter, he was still checked for "sharps" that he might use to hurt himself or others. He was asked more questions. Paul answered quickly, with some surprising answers.

How old are you?

"I'm five million years old."

Where are you from?

"I live on Mars."

Despite being hospitalized, Paul was found to be in a good mood, with a good memory, and "intellectual functioning that was above average. . . . Reasoning and judgment are not grossly impaired." His only other health issue was hypercholesterolemia, or high levels of cholesterol in the blood, which had been diagnosed three years earlier. He claimed to have a good relationship with his family, including being "very close to his father" and a supportive stepmother. He claimed to have a friend by the name of Joe Wise in Oklahoma City, although it wasn't clear if the friend existed.

His mental diagnosis was positive, considering his situation: schizophrenia, paranoid, in partial remission.

In what had to come as a shock to my father, Paul told the Griffin doctors that his goals were to "comply with treatment and realize his dreams of marriage." He said he'd had an ongoing relationship for the past fifteen years with a woman, and that he intended to marry Lynne when she finished her nursing degree. As for his plans, Paul said he would "wait for his girlfriend and possibly continue working until he retires." He listed his support system as his family, his "stable job," and "some support from his intended wife." But in yet another shock, I'm sure, for my father, Paul also told the doctors that he planned to move to Hennessey.

Paul was placed back on "chemotherapy," and then ordered to start taking Mellaril again, attend individual and group therapy, and attend classes to "obtain a better understanding of the pitfalls in stopping current medication." The latter was a class that our own father might have wanted to teach. As his stay continued, Paul began to reveal other details about his life. His hobbies, he said, were religion, reading, watching TV, and movies. He emphasized again how close he was to his family, and he reported having a good relationship with his girlfriend and other close friends.

"He always had a good relationship with his family," social worker Roy Williams wrote. "He has a history of a high level of functioning for the past several years. He has been able to hold a job with minimal difficulty. His father and stepmother are involved and supportive. He owns a mobile home near Guthrie which he can return to. He can also return to his job." However, another report warned:

> Mr. Hight has a long (history) of mental illness. (He) complains of auditory hallucinations and paranoid thinking. He is afraid he might kill himself or others.

The usual logs were kept of Paul's stay in Ward 53, and at some point, Paul did change his mind about moving to Hennessey. He would return to Guthrie. Dad took advantage of the improvement in Paul's health to leave town for a few days, only to return after a call from social worker Williams on June 12, 1989. Paul had been deemed stable and was ready to return home and to work. Dad picked him up at 1:00 p.m. Wednesday, June 14. On the car ride back to Guthrie, Paul was treated to one of Dad's infamous lectures—a flashback to his youth. When we were children, Dad's Sunday lectures could sting like a swarm of wasps. In this instance, he channeled his former Marine Corps drill sergeant.

"You have to take your medication, Paul. Can you do that?"

"I will."

"What happened this time?"

"I don't know. I think I can deal with it now. It makes me nervous. I don't like living in that home by myself."

"Well, you have to. I'm getting older and can't take care of you anymore. You have to take care of yourself. You have to take your medicine."

"I understand."

Paul had never admitted to the family that he suffered from mental illness, and he wasn't about to do so now. Nothing else was said on the trip. Arriving at Paul's house, father and son exchanged a quick good-bye.

Less than a month later, Paul attended the baptism of my first daughter, Elena, at our Edmond parish, although he did not play an active role in the ceremony at Saint John's. He seemed happy for Nan and me, especially when we took everyone out to lunch after the baptism—that never seemed to change, Paul always loved a good meal.

About that same time, Paul received a small monthly raise of $53.50, and records show he worked regularly for more than a year. Then illness and injuries began to cause him to miss days. Some absences could also have been because Paul still disliked, even resented, the colder days of outside winter work required of ODOT highway employees.

Then in 1990, Paul found himself in a similar situation to when he was a priest in Tulsa: His supervisor changed. The supportive Crabtree was gone, and his glowing evaluations of the past no longer mattered. "Paul has been off work with re-occurring health problems a lot in the past six months. Being off so much has prevented him from achieving his potential," one 1990 evaluation said. "Paul needs to spend more time on the job and be more observant to the work procedures going on around him. He needs to become more involved with his job and the crew." Unlike with his previous evaluations, Paul didn't deign to respond to the negative assessment of his new supervisor. That section was left blank, although Paul did sign the evaluation on Monday, June 25, 1990.

One has a sense that Paul knew his days at ODOT were numbered. Three weeks later, he was taken into protective custody again. Paul had quit taking his medication. He had returned to staring at the sky while at work. He had ignited a fire in his home by throwing lighted cigarettes into a trash can, where thankfully, the fire stayed. Documents from this period include interviews with Paul that questioned whether he was Catholic, with a question mark placed beside the word. "His parents and employers have both reported erratic and bizarre behavior," wrote J. David Gordon, an outpatient therapist at the Wheatland clinic in Guthrie. "He has become a danger to self in recent weeks."

Once again, the judge made a ruling. The documents were signed. Paul was evaluated and committed. July 17, 1990, Paul was taken back to Norman and placed in what was now known as Griffin Memorial Hospital. It was Paul's fourth time and, as one report would state, another of "multiple admissions to a mental health hospital." Reportedly, Paul said he didn't know why he was there except he couldn't concentrate at work. The prognosis, however, was the same: schizophrenia, paranoid type, although doctors didn't find paranoia this time. They did find his mental illness to be in "partial remission versus schizophrenia residual type." His medication was changed to 30 milligrams of the antipsychotic drug Loxitane before bedtime. Doctors determined Paul was now allergic to Thorazine, Stelazine, and Mellaril, the latter of which had kept him stable for longer periods. In another surprise, Paul told doctors he had "no active family support." That statement was listed as one of Paul's liabilities, along with the chronic state of his disease.

> [Patient] has no active psychotic symptoms, but he has been suffering from poor concentration, stares at the sky, amnesity (amnesia), and his job performance has decreased.

Paul had also learned the routine of being committed. He was calm and "cooperative, friendly, and willing to take his medication as prescribed." He denied he was depressed, suicidal, or had violent thoughts, and expressed concern about his job if he stayed hospitalized too long (he had learned that the hospital valued stable employment). Doctors told him that before he could be released, he would have to exhibit no possibility of returning to violent behavior. No more "bizarre behavior" either such as staring at the sky or sun, and he had to take his medication. They increased his dosage to 50 milligrams of Loxitane. A complete physical was ordered. Dr. Larry White, the resident psychiatrist, and Dr. H. L. Head, the medical director, handled that.

Now forty-seven, Paul had shrunk from almost six foot four inches to less than six foot two, more than an inch from his original height. He was considered moderately obese at 235 pounds. He continued to have high cholesterol. Other than that, he was physically normal, even remarkably healthy for his age. The doctors told Paul he would need to exercise more and regulate his diet. For Paul, that must have been an odd and difficult request. He walked regularly and worked outside, so why would he need more exercise? And as for cutting back his calories, food was one of the few reliable comforts my brother enjoyed in life.

The physical exam also revealed something startling—something that no one in the family, including Paul, seemed to know: Paul's left testicle had "severely atrophied" because of a case of mumps that the doctors believed had occurred in his twenties.

My sister Susan did recall later Paul being sent home from school for a period of time in his twenties. The cause: a bad virus spreading through the school's students and causing swelling of the glands. For most people, recovery from mumps is quick and without complications, but for someone whose genetics point to mental illness, mumps could have a secondary and more devastating effect. The Centers for Disease Control and the Mayo Clinic have reported that complications from mumps can lead to inflammation of the brain, and "encephalitis can lead to neurological problems and become life-threatening," according to the Mayo Clinic.

And that's not the only complication. Another possible side effect is "membranes and fluid around the brain and spinal cord," the Mayo Clinic reported. That condition, known as meningitis, can occur if the mumps virus spreads through one's bloodstream to infect the central nervous system. Studies dating to the late 1800s and 1930s also suggest links between viral infections such as mumps and schizophrenia and bipolar disorder. *The Psychiatric Times* reported that studies in the 1930s included experiments "in which cerebrospinal fluid . . . from patients with schizophrenia was injected into rabbit brains."

By the time Paul suffered from mumps, an effective vaccine had yet to be developed, and one would not be brought to market until 1968. When the mumps vaccination did become available, I didn't question Mom when she told me I needed to be vaccinated immediately. I didn't realize at the time that she might have been so insistent because of Paul's earlier bout with the disease, although I don't remember anything being said.

Elena Conis wrote in *Vaccine Nation: America's Changing Relationship with Immunization*:

> When [the mumps] struck teens and adults, its usually rare complications—including inflammation of the reproductive organs and pancreas—become more frequent and more troublesome.

Another analysis of several studies, released in 2012, further supports the possibility of a link between mumps and subsequent mental illness. Meta-analysis of seven studies of 2,424 cases shows that "viral infection was associated with nearly two-fold increase of adult nonaffective psychosis." Separate meta-analysis of 1,035 cases of "childhood . . . infections, particularly viral infections, may be associated with a nearly two-fold risk of adult schizophrenia." And the "mumps infection was reported to be associated with increased risk of nonaffective psychosis. . . . It has been reported that certain genotypes of the mumps's virus (type C and D) exhibit greater neurovirulence than others."

In other words, certain strains of the mumps's virus have a greater chance of affecting the nervous system. "Mumps have been reported to be associated with long-term difficulties with memory and other neurological (issues) in humans."

Could a bad case of the mumps be what led to Paul's paranoid schizophrenia? Could it have been the mumps and not LSD, as Daddy had always said, that caused the sudden chemical imbalance in my brother's brain? In hindsight, was the fact that Paul had never shown even the slightest hint of mental illness before coming down with the mumps be because he did not become vulnerable until after having the mumps? A few years later, Paul would start to suffer from catatonic states and mental illness. Could the mumps have been the mechanism? He had suffered a severe form of it, serious enough to shrivel one of his testicles? Had school officials known but not made my parents aware of the latter?

His 1990 physical revealed he suffered from mumps, but doctors merely noted it in passing. They did this despite the studies and historical connections between mumps and mental illness known by then. Because no further studies followed, Paul and his family would never know for sure what had caused his mental illness beyond some possible genetic link. All would live in fear that they or their children or grandchildren might suffer the same fate in life.

At the time, with his mental condition improving, Paul was scheduled to be discharged nine days later on July 26, 1990. But it's unclear exactly when Paul was released. His complete physical was conducted and signed on July 30. On July 31, a discharge plan that stated he would return home by bus and follow up with treatment at the Wheatland clinic. A final discharge was signed on August 8 and August 9. "The patient was moved into the ward and quickly adjusted and rapidly given lobby and grounds [access] . . . which he dealt with appropriately," the release report said. "Mr. Hight stabilized very quickly, and it was felt his job might be in jeopardy if he continued to be off. Due to his improved status, I decided to allow his discharge."

The part about his job being in jeopardy was correct.

JOE HIGHT

August 10, 1990, Paul filled out an application for "vested benefits" from ODOT. He had used all his sick leave. The application stated that Paul had worked seven years and six months of "credited service, and I wish to be elected a vested benefit in the retirement system" with the state. He asked to retain his health and dental insurance.

A letter dated August 16 from Dr. Harold A. McGuffey, a psychiatrist at Wheatland, stated that Paul had "been removed from his current duties with the Department of Transportation due to safety concerns related to his mental and physical condition. . . . It is possible that his current status precludes his ability to perform job duties competently and safely. This letter supports the claim he needs to make for disability."

Nine days later, Paul sent a letter asking for a leave of absence without pay "during my recovery period."

He would never return to work again.

On October 17, 1990, he received his last paycheck of $1,185.83 from the state. Three words written in green ink simply note "payroll removal—resigned." He was not yet forty-eight years old, but he was now on long-term disability. Whether that was a blessing or a curse remained to be seen.

As the fall days turned colder that year, Paul was initially elated that he didn't have to return to work in such conditions and was no longer on call when ice or snow struck the state. He was free to stay inside his warm mobile home, watch TV, read his Bible, debate those who dared knock on his door, go to restaurants when someone asked, and enjoy his walks. He did not have much money because he kept giving it away, but then again, he didn't care about money anyway. He had a home that wouldn't be taken away and now the time to make the long round trip to visit Lynne in Checotah. After suffering for so many years, after losing the calling he had loved so much, he had a second chance and the time to craft a life to suit him.

If he took his medicine. If he took his medicine. If . . .

Chapter 18

Tormented Notes of Hierarchy

Dad and I walked slowly up the concrete steps to the front door of Paul's mobile home in east Guthrie. It was a mild, somewhat chilly spring evening that April 5, 1991. The previous day, Paul had been taken to Griffin Memorial Hospital for the fifth time, the third time in two years. His refusal to take his oral medicine had become a severe problem, so much so that doctors had started giving him injections of 100 milligrams of the antipsychotic Haldol, or haloperidol. Despite having received a shot only five days before, Paul was claiming that he was hearing voices.

He was also becoming paranoid.

"The angels are talking to me."

"Julius Caesar is telling me what to do."

"I'm hearing King David's voice."

"I'm scared of what they're saying."

The voices scared Paul enough that my brother sought treatment. He said the Haldol, known for causing anxiety, among other side effects, was making him paranoid. In the early 1990s, doctors rarely gave people suffering from schizophrenia monthly injections, despite the drug being less expensive than other medications and suitable for someone such as Paul on Social Security disability. For one, the injections, although given in the buttocks, can be painful, and the side effects can include anxiety. Haldol is also not recommended for older patients with a history of dementia or heart disease. Given that Mom had died of a heart attack and Paul had high cholesterol, Haldol seemed a strange choice for him. But then, with Paul refusing to take his oral medicine, the doctors didn't have many options. Haldol injections should be supplemented by oral dosages, later studies would show, but it's unclear whether Paul was receiving the latter. No one in the Hight family, perhaps not even Dad, knew exactly what was occurring with Paul's treatment by then.

A new round of hospitalizations started in March 1991 with Paul's admittance to the Oklahoma County Crisis Intervention Center in Oklahoma City. OCCIC was one of several adult crisis centers in Oklahoma that provided emergency services for adults with mental health, substance abuse, or co-occurring issues. Patients weren't supposed to stay more than three days, but Paul remained there for three weeks, from March 14, 1991, to April 4, 1991, until being transferred to Griffin Memorial for further treatment.

Paul reported feeling much better after taking 50 milligrams of Mellaril at Griffin Memorial, even though he was apparently allergic to it, or at least so doctors had previously thought. The inconsistencies were consistent with this visit and previous ones. This time, after Paul had committed himself, Dad asked me to go with him to Paul's house. We entered the home to the overwhelming but familiar odor of stale cigarettes, some of which emanated from an ashtray overflowing with cigarette butts on the small table where Paul kept his Bible and the notepad he used to scribble down his thoughts. The small kitchen was cluttered with dirty dishes and pans crusted with days-old food. The refrigerator was all but empty.

Dad shook his head in disgust and told me to stay put while he went to get something from Paul's bedroom at the far end of the mobile home. As I waited, my eyes returned to Paul's notepad, and being curious, I picked it up. What I saw befuddled me. Instead of notes to himself or a short grocery list, Paul had scrawled a diagram, a stack of semicircles from the looks of it. The smallest semicircle was at the bottom of the page and the largest at the top. It was a hierarchy of some sort, and a rough, somewhat jagged line was drawn vertically through the center of the semicircles from top to bottom. I noticed that the semicircles also contained names in the form of a disconcerting sentence. To my surprise, my name was on the first line:

I am Joe Hight, and I rule over him.
I am Wilber Hight, and I rule over the Hights.
I am the mayor, and I rule over Guthrie.
I am Governor David Walters, and I rule over Oklahoma.
I am George Bush, and I rule over my country.

Then in a strange twist, the names began to change from politicians and people he knew to celebrities. Bryant Gumbel and Jane Pauley were ruling or had ruled the networks as hosts of the *Today Show*. He was either a fan of the two or the show or had watched it one time, perhaps when he had been in the hospital ward. In Paul's altered state of reality, Gumbel and Pauley had made an impression on him because he also included them in his chain of command:

I am Jane Pauley, and I rule over the TV networks.
I am Bryant Gumbel, and I rule over the air waves (sic).

Then the focus changed to the religious icons of his upbringing:

I am Mary, and I rule over people's hearts.
I am Paul, and I rule over people's words.
I am Satan, and I rule over the earth.

The reference to Satan recalled Paul's frightening vision of the devil trying to lure him into hell and the angel who had come afterward to

191

reassure him of God's glory all those years ago in the Tulsa rectory. As I read, I could feel my brother returning to that moment, only this time, he had transformed himself into a deity.

> *I am Jesus, and I rule over the universe.*
> *I AM GOD, AND I RULE OVER THE HEAVENS!*

The letters in all caps and the exclamation mark graced the top of the page, ending the diagram. My mind returned to another time, our family kitchen, the day my brother approached me with a knife clutched in his hand. Had the voices commanded him that I was a threat to him and them? Had they decided that I needed to be destroyed? I turned to the next page. The words flew at me:

> *FUCK, SHIT, DAMN. . . .*

The words were in all caps, repeated over and over. Despite future studies that would show cursing can be a sign of great intelligence, profanity at the time was taboo, especially in my mother's staunchly Catholic home. But there the words were, written in a variety of ways as well as in all caps, with or without exclamation points, as if Paul were trying to define or defuse or embolden the meaning of the four-letter words by writing them in different ways. I had never heard my brother utter even a casual *damn*, so it was stunning to see them in his own handwriting. Surely not, I thought, trying to convince myself that the handwriting was not his, but I recognized the swift strokes, the letters flowing together, as clearly being Paul's.

My father's voice startled me back to reality.

"Joe, we need to go!"

Jumping to my feet, I blurted, "Daddy, I found this notepad. You need to see it."

I handed over the notepad and watched as Dad studied the pages. He grimaced but didn't say a word. Instead, he tucked the notepad under his arm and motioned for me to go.

I regretted reading only the first two pages. Who knows what the other pages might have revealed about my brother's troubled mind. Years later, I would find more such writings among the few possessions Paul left behind—tucked in a folder, an envelope, a box—anywhere that could hold them, eerily reminiscent of what Mom used to do with money and the clippings about Linda's death.

Paul's writing covered college-ruled notebooks, green legal pads, junk mail, and credit-card or bank statements. Some of the writings would make you smile. Some would make you laugh. Some would make you blush. Some were spiritual. Others, inspiring. Many, puzzling. Certain words at times were obscured by cigarette burns. Water spills and drink stains warped many other screeds.

All smelled as if Paul had been smoking heavily as he wrote. Overall, the writings—deeply emotional statements and unintelligible gibberish—illuminated the fine line between lunacy and enlightenment. In certain instances, Paul's mind appeared to have created a language only he could translate. Or maybe a language that only God could understand.

Reading them could be both frightening and hurtful. I didn't know whether to be flattered or scared if I came across my name. Everybody mentioned seemed to have played an important role in his life or have been loathed for that role. One page was covered with odd writing and confusing words on the top and bottom and read:

> *My Plan—To have a life … Joy & Love through*
> *kindness to others.*

On another, Paul wrote what amounted to a poem about his own mind's battle with demons:

> *Temperance????*
> *… keenly to faith*
> *Righteous is under the law*
> *for the kingdom of God*
> *Soul, body & Prosperity*

After a full page outlining his budget needs, he then wrote: "Court case 1267," circling all of the numbers, and then:

> *1. Repentance*
>   *Turning from sin to virtue.*
>   *(For the kingdom)*
>   *Careful practice of the commandments*
> *2. Baptism & Being Born Again*
>   *Being Saved.*
> *3. Persistence in Faith [Gospel}*
> *4. End—Salvation.*

Under an entry entitled accounting notes, he tried to figure out a budget while he was trying to figure out God, along with his and others' places in life. Our father was constantly listed as a "technical adviser" or by other titles or just his name. Paul consistently listed his name beside or above Dad's as "Paul W. Hight." Another page contained a series of phone numbers and names with more about his spirituality.

> *Ask and you shall receive. Just Be thankful. . . . Jesus died for my sins & resurrected to give Life. I accepted Him as the Lord.*

That was followed by a series of calculations in which Paul seemed calculate the points required for true salvation. Do you get fifty points for miracles? Twenty-five points for wisdom? Other points for condolence? And more for speaking in tongues and interpretation of them? My brother's mind was seemingly trying to figure out his past while charting a course for the future. He wrote about knowledge, about the "wisdom in discourse," about having faith in miracles and healing, about the "disconnect of spirits," about speaking in tongues and the interpretation of them, and about prophecy.

He wrote words that seemed to hold meaning for him: love, joy, peace, mildness, self-centered charity, kindness, self-control, patience, and long-suffering, the latter a reference to his own long, desperate battle with mental illness. He wrote budget numbers. He wrote "Food $100" in red—followed by "All the various Suffering (Salvation) & Poverty & Death are far illusions in the mind. They slet [sic] in the heart," signed, in his handwriting, by Francis Frankford Jr.

Paul's notes provide insight into what his daily life entailed or maybe what he wanted it to be.

On one page, he made a routine:

> *1. Lift weights & exercise.*
> *2. Talk to demons in a loving way.*
> *3. Smoke cigarettes.*
> *4. Drink Pop.*
> *5. Call Mary & Father & Ruth & Marcel.*
> *6. Clean up living Room & Kitchen.*
> *7. Read Daily Blessing & study the Bible.*
> *8. Speak tongues & interpret.*
> *9. Prophecy.*
> *10. Clean up bedroom.*

On another, a note to self reminded him that he needed to eat "real meat," vegetables, and starch. He made a list of important vitamins and the need for a "protein drink."

He set personal goals:

> *1. Give up Alcohol.*
> *2. Keep Personal Hygiene (in) Public*
>   *1. Brush teeth and tongue.*
>   *2. Showering once a day.*
>   *3. Wash hair every other day.*
>   *4. Cleaning my gentalia adequately.*
>   *5. Picking up everyday & having publicly kept house.*
>   *6. Having P???? .... After cleaning at 11:00 ....????*
>   *7. Get up at 5:15 a.m. early ... 10 yrs (68).*

As Paul's mind became more and more lost in the interior voices, tasks such as cleaning would fall off the lists. In their place, he took to writing notes to the named voices in his head:

Dear Pacilli, Heard your reply—yes. Paul

He appeared fascinated with or maybe tormented by names and his place within those names. Page after notebook page, Paul wrote name after name, sometimes using his name in a series of names with different middle and last names, sometimes with his own name, sometimes with those of "Wilber," or as he sometimes would spell it, "Wilbur." Then he would write Mom's name repeatedly. On occasion, he would include the names of celebrities. Long before the presidential election of 2016, he wrote Samuel Trump, Ivanka Trump, and then Donald Trump. Hillary Clinton was placed on another page among a series of names that included his own.

Sometimes lucidity would suddenly return. Incoherent ramblings returned to budget figures as he tried to track his credit-card bills, rent, food, and other items. His diet changed as well. Food was listed as only $40, although he listed $100 for pop and $75 for cigarettes. He had a $45 allowance for unknown reasons. He left only $15 in "surplus."

On another, a coffee spill washes like a wave on a beach, discoloring different places on the page. Just as quickly, the whole tone of the writing changes as if the wave had swept over Paul, and the names start again. The abrupt change is stark. The contrast is startling. In one, he uses comedian Jerry Lewis's name:

Jerry Lewis Robinson Graham
Jerry Lewis Graham Marshall Grant
Jerry Lou Robinson Grant
Jerry Lou Robinson
Jerry Lewis Graham Roberts
Jerry Lewis Graham
Marshal

Director
Jerry Lewis Graham
Otto
Robinson

He also lists possible occupations he might pursue.

1. Accounting. 2. Paralegal. 3. Computer Science.

He then changed his mind and wrote:

1. Psychiatrist. 2. Priest. 3. Counselor. 4. Politician. 5. Businessman. 6. Accountant. 7. Lawyer. 8. Mechanic. 9. Technician.

If possible economically take all 3 courses of accounting, law & mechanics as well as General medicine & psychiatry through Jesus, Holy Spirit, and Me. Rather than for the Institute which is a bit corrupt in its handling of the subject of Law & Accounting as well as mechanic joke.
Better than anybody's ever done.

After all this, Paul declared that he would become "a general practitioner, in order of psychiatrist."

Some entries indicate that Paul was still trying to rationalize how his vocation in life had taken such a wrong turn. However, the reality was that my brother was drifting deeper into an unrealistic state as he next began to give himself titles. After declaring in public that he was Julius Caesar and King David, Paul was taken to Griffin Memorial again.

That trip again created about as many inconsistencies as his writing. Paul went through another complete physical—this time while "wearing multiple shirts"—as well as more psychiatric assessments. Paul knew the routine by now, and thus maybe how to work it: Get stabilized and get out as quickly as possible.

His desire to leave was understandable, considering what patients were going through then at the hospital. Paul himself was in the throes of a change. He told the doctors that he no longer wanted to return to Guthrie or even Hennessey but to Bethany, which would be a return to his teenage years when he first began his journey to the priesthood. Paul had also become convinced that the voices were making him sick, not the medications the doctors were giving him.

Dr. Suk J. Han confirmed this:

> The patient becomes sick with paranoid thinking and auditory hallucinations, and symptoms have not improved with outpatient treatment and the short period of OCCIC treatment. . . . Patient reports he feels better already. However, it is questionable whether symptoms have improved due to Haloperidol or Mellaril.

Paul then underwent another complete, more invasive physical that included determining whether the foreskin on his penis retracted easily, according to his file. In another turnaround, the physical revealed that he had no allergies, even though previous physicals had indicated that Paul had multiple allergies associated with his medication. The physical also found that he suffered from bronchitis.

The doctors noted that his left testicle had atrophied "by history," again alluding to what is now called "childhood mumps." Paul had cigarette burns on his left forearm as if he had been trying to extinguish cigarettes on himself.

A note stated that Paul requested that he not be given another rectal exam because he had recently received one at the Oklahoma County Crisis Intervention Center and "was reported to be normal." The physical also revealed that Paul was complaining of "occasional rectal soreness," but nothing more was noted, questioned, followed up on, or investigated.

According to the report, Paul told the doctors that he had begun to smoke in 1974, about the time he was being forced to resign from the priesthood. He said he drank one can of beer a month, but he had not used any other alcohol or narcotic. He said he wore "photo gray lenses" and admitted for the first time that he had "sustained retinal damage from looking directly at the sun for extended periods of time."

Paul was stabilized quickly, but a report filed April 4 by Carol L. Crossover—after talking to Dad and David Gordon of the Wheatland clinic—seems to indicate my brother's condition had worsened:

> The patient has not functioned very well for the last year. He has been able to maintain in the community on a marginal level for the last year. He has been at OCCIC several times since his last discharge. He apparently has been exhibiting some 'dark moods.' He withdraws into his mobile home and does not want to see anyone, including his family. He will sometimes go out at night. . . . He has also been telling a close married female friend of the family that he loved her, which is completely out of character for him.

Despite the new issues of concern, Crossover added:

> The patient will require close observation and evaluation of his chemotherapy needs. He also needs to exhibit appropriate interactions with others. His family and friends are involved and supportive of him. He will be able to return to his mobile home in Guthrie when ready for discharge. It seems unlikely that he will require any long-term inpatient treatment. He will be referred back to Wheatland services with a recommendation for involvement in day activities.

Four days later, the now forty-eight-year-old Paul signed his "participation in the discharge planning process," allowing his return to his Guthrie home.

He was released for the last time from Griffin Memorial Hospital. His now supportive family lived within driving distance, his discharge papers said, and friends of the family would try to help watch him as well. A new friend had also resurfaced, one who understood the priesthood and sympathized with Paul much more than Dad. And Paul's rekindled relationship with Lynne was pointing toward marriage—if his deteriorating mental health did not deter their plans.

Chapter 19

The Rage Inside

Except for his Irish brogue and balding head, Father Denis Hanrahan and my brother Paul were alike in many ways. Both knew early in life that they were going to be priests. Both came from big Catholic families that encouraged them. Both were known for their kindness and wit. Both had deep Irish roots, although Hanrahan's ran much deeper. Both wore big, black-rimmed glasses behind which were found particularly arresting eyes. Both had stooped postures at times. Both could be instantly friendly to anyone and could talk about the Bible as if they had written it.

Yet they had their differences too. Hanrahan was born in Dublin, Ireland, in 1935, seven years before Paul, and ordained in 1959. He liked to talk about how he grew up in a parish in which twenty young men became priests, a point of pride for the close-knit Irish Catholic community. His older brother, Michael, also became a priest, and the Hanrahan brothers both ended up not only in the United States but also in Oklahoma.

After Father Elmer Robnett died in March 1990, Hanrahan took Robnett's place as pastor of our old family parish in 1991; his brother died that same year. He remained at Saint Mary's the rest of his priestly

career. Not too long after Hanrahan's arrival in Guthrie, he heard that
a former priest was living east of town, although how he discovered it
remains unknown. Many years had passed since anyone connected to
the priesthood had attempted to reach out to Paul. Hanrahan did so
without hesitation.

Maybe sensing a kindred spirit, Paul let the Irishman in. The two
men found that they shared a fondness for discussion, especially about
the Bible and faith. One of Hanrahan's strongest beliefs was that suffering on earth would earn a soul a crown in heaven. Paul liked hearing
that. Before long, my brother was telling people about his new priest
friend from Guthrie, one with whom he could discuss anything.

Hanrahan had made a friend too. "[Paul] was a kind, nice man,"
Hanrahan would say later. "I enjoyed our visits. I was very comfortable
with him. He was my friend."

Indeed, Hanrahan became a regular visitor at Paul's, going so far
as to take my brother once a month to what the Irish priest called "the
smoke shop" for cheap cigarettes. The two of them also liked to do
lunch, often frequenting Mazzio's for its all-you-can-eat pizza buffet in
nearby Edmond or Oklahoma City. Hanrahan liked pizza well enough,
but Paul's appetite for it was the kind that made those who offer buffets
tremble—not to mention that Paul put away breadsticks like potato
chips. Hanrahan would occasionally ask Paul, "How can you put away
so many of those breadsticks? I can't hold a candle to you." Paul would
just give Hanrahan a big smile before popping another one into his
mouth.

Occasionally, Paul's past with the Church they both loved would
come up, and Hanrahan came to believe that Paul had been pushed
into laicization by the Tulsa diocese. Like a counselor would a patient
or a priest would a parishioner in the confessional, Hanrahan assured
Paul that he would keep in confidence whatever Paul might want to
say about what had happened to him during that process. He gave my
brother an opening in which Paul could have said anything about any
priest, any bishop, anyone against whom he carried a grudge for what
had happened to him. Paul had nary a word to say.

"He never said a bad word about anyone. Never had a chip on his shoulder. Never a mean attitude," Father Hanrahan said. "Paul seemed to like most of the priests and bishops."

Likely because of Hanrahan's warm, welcoming nature, Paul started to attend Mass at Saint Mary's again. However, he still did not return to his family's old front pew but to one in the back three rows. Some people might say he did not want to upset those parishioners who did not want a former priest in their midst. Others might say he did so to reduce his anxiety about being out and amongst people. And a few men and women, those prone to frequenting the back rows of Catholic churches themselves, might say Paul did so because he felt unworthy to sit any farther forward. I do not know what caused my brother to seek out the back rows in his old family church, just that he did so this time as he had the last. Surprisingly, however, Paul did not flee at the end of Mass as he had previous times. Instead, he lingered afterward to visit with his fellow parishioners and Father Hanrahan. My brother's return was proof of the difference one kind person can make in whether a person with mental illness is shunned or embraced.

Although Paul and Father Hanrahan held each other in mutual esteem, they had their differences too. Hanrahan soon learned that, as he described it, "Paul was such a sucker for a sad story." Seeing people take advantage of his friend bothered Hanrahan and, as so many others had before him, the priest advised Paul to be more careful with his money. In the end they agreed to disagree. Paul would never accept that his need for his money was greater than those who asked for it. And Paul carried that belief all his life.

Looking back, it would seem to have been a relatively happy time for Paul, certainly one of his most engaged since leaving the priesthood. But no one knows, except for Paul, what he dealt with on any given day or hour or minute. There are twenty-four hours in a day, 1,440 minutes, and 86,400 seconds. As a cradle Catholic who attended Catholic schools and minor seminary, Paul would have been taught to consider each and every moment as an opportunity to do good or evil or nothing—the latter being a sin of apathy. Catholics don't just worry about telling lies—they worry about sins of omission, the lie of not telling the whole truth. Alone in his home with only his mind or even in the stray moments while out and about with others, what thoughts, emotions, cravings, pains, and voices did my brother battle? That was something none of us, no matter how much we loved him, or how many questions we asked him, could ever know.

Paul, himself, had vowed never to return to Griffin Memorial, and he did what he could to ensure that wouldn't happen. He religiously showed up for his monthly shots at the Wheatland clinic, which helped him maintain the stability needed to remain on the outside and at home. He continued to suffer, however, from the medication's side effects. Still, he could pull himself together when people came to visit, and he looked forward to when our brother Bill came to stay. Mostly, though, Paul stayed at home, content to spend his time testing his biblical knowledge against the televangelists and scoffing at those who encouraged their followers to touch the screen and be healed.

With his mental illness seemingly somewhat in check, Paul lived a simple life but not necessarily a solitary one. When he wasn't watching TV, Paul was calling people or they were calling him, including all his brothers and sisters. Paul called our house at least once a week to ask about my job, now at the state's largest newspaper, *The Oklahoman*, or how Elena and Nan were doing. He was excited when he heard Nan was pregnant with our second child in 1993 and thrilled when Elyse was born that December. Nan and I decided this dear older brother and former priest who now was doing so well would be the perfect godfather for our Elyse. Paul laughed when I asked him, only to quickly turn serious and proclaim himself honored when he realized I wasn't kidding. We asked our oldest niece, Linda, now an emergency room nurse and named for the aunt whom her mother, Susan, never knew, to be Elyse's godmother. At the baptism, I felt my sister Linda's presence as the cold water was poured over Elyse's tiny head, and everybody chuckled as the baby let out a shriek.

Back in Guthrie, Paul was making new friends at church and had taken to calling them as well. Mary Wheeler was one with whom he spoke almost daily. She recalled that Paul, in a recurring theme of his life, liked to talk about restaurants, so they often exchanged reviews of various establishments they had been to from Red Lobster to Steak and Ale. Wheeler once sent a note to Paul in which she wrote:

> *I want to take the opportunity to let you know I care about you and enjoy the phone calls so much. I hope we can remain friends for many years to come.*

Paul had shown he could develop friendships with some depth, and although he rarely mentioned a love interest to anyone, Paul had continued to dream about marriage—more specifically marrying Lynne. In his early fifties now, Paul showed no awareness that time might be running out on this. Still, the possibility seemed remote. If anyone asked about Lynne, he would say either that she was a girlfriend or he planned to marry her. His pledge to never return to Griffin Memorial, however, seemed to renew his efforts to reach out to Lynne. He called her when he could afford to and borrowed Father Hanrahan's old Subaru to make the drive to rural Chouteau to visit when he could.

Lynne and Paul had met nearly two decades ago and had been dating since the late 1970s, but only Lynne could answer how determined she was to marry Paul, especially considering his personal and professional setbacks. Family members remember her making the drive to Guthrie only once to see Paul, and they recalled the visit as more akin to one from a friend than a romantic encounter. Maybe Paul misinterpreted a caring friendship as love. Maybe Lynne worried about whether his stability was solid enough to hold up under marriage.

No one in the Hight family seems to recall ever seeing them hug, let alone kiss, although that could easily be explained by a shyness with regard to public displays of affection or a reluctance on Paul's part rooted in the vow of celibacy he had made some thirty years before as a priest. After all, what did we know anyway? Does anyone profess to understand exactly what brings couples together or tears them apart, much less what happens between them or behind closed doors?

Lynne also had her own personal challenges, including a son in his thirties with emotional and mental issues who still lived at home. That might explain Lynne's soft heart when it came to Paul and her willingness to love him without putting the demands on him that usually come with a relationship. As the months and years passed into early 1995, Paul seemed to also become more uncertain about whether Lynne wanted to marry him or what their future held. He started to ease away when asked how Lynne was doing or, when forced to answer, simply said that she was doing okay.

Then April 19, 1995, upended all of our worlds.

That morning Gulf War veteran Timothy McVeigh and his coconspirator Terry Nichols carried out a right-wing extremist plot against the United States government to coincide with the anniversary of the final day of the 1993 fifty-one-day FBI siege at Waco, Texas. McVeigh parked a yellow Ryder rental van in front of the Alfred P. Murrah Federal Building in downtown Oklahoma City. At 9:02 a.m., the truck exploded, creating a cavity that stretched the length and width of the almost block-wide building. Anyone walking near the building at that point was vaporized. The explosion rocked the city, causing nearby buildings to collapse and shattering windows twenty blocks away; the blast was felt all the way to Guthrie. Seven miles to the north, I was working as community editor at *The Daily Oklahoman* in a twelve-story tower built to withstand winds of three hundred miles per hour because of the state's location in Tornado Alley. The bomb blast spread like a tsunami wave to the north, and soon *The Daily Oklahoman* tower swayed as if it were wheat in a strong Oklahoma wind. I looked out to see a massive gray cloud rising into the sky above downtown. For a moment, everything went silent and seemed to move in slow motion.

The world stopped to take a breath.

Then the phones started to ring.

By the time it was all over, 168 people, including nineteen children in an on-site day care and one nurse who ran to help, were dead. Hundreds had been injured. I worked for three months straight with few days off; after that, the bombing never strayed far from my mind. Media worldwide converged on the site of the worst domestic terrorist act in the country's history. Oklahoma City and Oklahoma would never be the same again. For years afterward, I could not recall what had happened before April 19 and 1994, the first full year of Elyse's life.

Two days later, Paul's world would be upended again.

* * * * *

On Friday night, April 21, 1995, then thirty-five-year-old Joe Mendosa climbed the stairs to the second-floor of the rural Chouteau home where his mother slept and beat her to death with a claw hammer. Earlier in the day, his mother had given him the weekly shot to control his mental illness. He thought she was trying to poison him.

Three days later, family members found the body of fifty-four-year-old Janet Lynne Brown—Paul's dear Lynne—wrapped in a carpet in that same bedroom.

The Associated Press wrote only four paragraphs about the murder. Nearly a year later, Mendosa pled guilty to first-degree murder. According to Assistant Mayes County District Attorney Chuck Ramsey, Mendosa did not want to put his family through a trial: "He said he did it, and he just wanted to get it over with." Mendosa's tape-recorded confession was played at his preliminary hearing. He was given life without parole.

On learning of Lynne's death, Paul entered another level of personal hell. The priesthood, which he had trained for and loved, had been taken from him. Now the woman he loved and had planned to marry had been taken from him. In his grief, whether Paul turned to his God in prayer is not known, but my brother appeared to receive some comfort in the companionship of a tan-colored mutt that friends began to see Paul with on his daily walks. No one in the family knew where the dog had come from; Paul, it seems, never said. Dad had earlier tried to help in Paul's time of sorrow by giving his son a guitar in the hope that Paul might find comfort in the music he once loved. But the next time Dad checked, Paul had given the guitar away. Someone needed it more.

No one seems to know if Paul was taking his medication, but from all appearances, he was not doing well. Records show that Paul filled out paperwork at Wheatland clinic, where he still went monthly for his shot and checkups, on July 1, 1995, and a discharge form, from Wheatland dated January 1, 1996. Father Hanrahan became deeply concerned about Paul's deteriorating mental health. He called Dad, now nearly eighty years old.

"[Your father] said he had done everything he could," Hanrahan recalled. "Paul was not his problem anymore."

One Hight family friend had witnessed the decline of Dad's relationship with his oldest son. Mary Welch worked at the Sinclair station Paul favored; her home was next door. She and her husband, Paul, were both close friends of Mom and Dad and knew my siblings and me. They considered themselves close friends of Paul's too. "[Your father] tried to do everything he could. He wasn't capable of doing it anymore. He didn't know how," said Mary, whose gentle eyes could disarm any unpleasant thought. "He was scared of Paul. Paul threatened him and wouldn't let him into his life."

Dad had related a unsettling encounter with Paul at the Sinclair station. My stepmother, Joy, was with him and recalled that they had driven to Guthrie to see Paul but found him on foot, headed to the gas station and talking loudly to himself. They pulled into the station's entrance; Paul spotted them and headed briskly toward the car. Dad was getting out to greet him, but before he could get more than a foot on the ground, Paul was standing over him. Summoning the most commanding voice he could muster at his age, Dad shouted: "Paul!"

"What do you want?" Paul asked.

"I know you're off. You need to take your medication."

"You leave me alone! Leave me alone or you'll regret it!" Paul yelled angrily, and with that, Paul grabbed the car door, slammed the door on Dad's leg, and stalked away without another word.

Dad's leg was bruised in the encounter, and his will for dealing with Paul's mental illness evaporated into nothingness, like gas fumes from the station's pumps. He feared Paul more than ever, and he no longer had the energy to try to monitor or fix Paul. As for his love and concern for his oldest son, that had not abated.

Not long afterward, Dad created the Paul W. Hight 1996 Revocable Living Trust Agreement. He named Paul as the beneficiary and me as trustee. Dad set aside $10,000 to benefit Paul if our father should die first. Any moneys from the trust would go to Paul as needed while Paul was alive and for funeral expenses when he died.

To Dad, that possibility seemed inevitable. "I can't do anything else," Dad told me. "I'm tired of dealing with this. I'm just getting too old. You may need to help me."

After the incident with Dad at the station, no one could reach Paul by phone, as far as we could tell. We heard about him mostly through sightings by family friends in Guthrie. He had taken to walking along State Highway 33 day and night, usually talking loudly to no one and shaking his fists in the air as if a swarm of wasps were stinging every corner of his mind. From what people described, the demons and the voices had intensified their assaults on my brother.

Paul was also visiting the Sinclair gas station five or six times a day. But this was not the Paul we knew, the friendly fellow who liked to linger and visit, but a sullen man who bought his pop and cigarettes fast and left without saying a word. And those were the good days. On others, Paul would mock the station's employees, calling them names—"superman," "the president," or "Spock" from the TV show *Star Trek*.

Paul was now frequenting other Guthrie businesses too, walking nearly a mile to the Treasure Mart in town, where police were called after Paul asked a clerk if he were a doorman and started to talk loudly to himself. Another time, Paul refused to come out of the mart's restroom but managed to leave before a police officer could arrive.

Paul was also no longer paying for his purchases with cash. Instead, he was writing small checks, most for about two dollars but never for more than ten. The checks kept bouncing, because Paul no longer had enough funds in the bank to cover them. Although Dad continued to receive and make phone calls about Paul, now I was receiving them as well. In late March 1996, Toni Daves, a bank employee and part-time police officer, called me at work about the matter. I asked him to call the sheriff and have Paul taken to a crisis center.

A few days later, Paul called Guthrie Federal Savings.

"Someone is stealing money from my account!" he yelled at the bank officer. "I want my account closed now!"

The bank refunded all the service charges Paul had incurred from the matter and issued him a check for his Social Security deposit, and then the bank closed his account. Paul no longer had a bank account.

The dog that had adopted him had disappeared.

Paul's car was gone too or perhaps he had given it away.

Sheriff Burris had left.

And so as had happened in Tulsa when this all begun and later at ODOT, there was no longer a friendly advocate in authority to take Paul to a crisis center in his time of need. Despite repeated phone calls from Dad, the new sheriff never responded. In his agitated state, Paul likely wouldn't have wanted that anyway.

At this time, no one was checking on Paul—not Dad, not friends, not law enforcement—because everyone feared him or feared what they might find if they did. Paul's gentle personality had turned into that of a bully, and a mean one at that. My brother no longer seemed able to bear the pain of life, and this change can be seen in his writings, as Paul tried to soothe his tortured mind. He struggled to understand what God wanted from him:

> *1. How does one love God?*
> *A. By keeping his commandment as interpreted by Jesus, Holy Spirit, and the Church.*
> *B. By maneuvering to God's needs through prayers of praise & thanksgiving, by giving to his Church, and by ministering to the needs of his people.*
> *C. By kissing Him on the cheek.*
> *D. By financing Him personally.*
> *E. By prayer & by telling Him we love Him.*
> *F. By being Good to yourself & being Good to others.*

G. By trying to understand his Position.
H. By looking at his read & being sintered in attitude
& behavior (limitation).
I. By taking rebuke & Christianity patiently &
responding in a positive & loving manner.

With Paul off his medication, the voices burned through his thoughts, demanding answers, seeking control. What Paul would have considered blasphemy when he was of sound mind became reality in the wounded one. He scribbled a final sentence to his list of what God wanted from him:

Summary: God is a S.O.B. ... & hates you a lot but
He expects you to still Love Him back!

Paul's mind had broken. His body became the voices' tool. Down went the notepad. Paul grabbed a kitchen chair and stomped out the front door, leaving the house open behind him. He hurled the chair over the well near the creek. He headed along State Highway 33 back to the Sinclair gas station.

It was early evening on Saturday, April 6, 1996, almost a year since Lynne had been murdered. Mary Welch was behind the counter at the service station. Paul had already visited the station several times that day. During one trip, he had brought his mail with him, only to tear it up and toss it in a trash can before departing. Knowing Paul had been having issues, Mary had checked the trash and found a check from Guthrie Federal Savings made out to Paul for several hundred dollars; she would make sure Dad received it. On this trip, Paul was still in jeans, wearing a black leather jacket and a ball cap.

Looking closer, Mary noticed that he was dirty and looked as if he hadn't washed for several days. The sun was beginning to set. Traffic was heavy on the nearby Interstate 35, and a steady stream of customers was keeping Mary busy. "Cars were everywhere," Mary recalled, but in a brief lull, she spotted Paul through the windows, stomping toward the station like an angry bull. Mary had no way of knowing, but the voices were taunting Paul again, driving him forward like a car that only they could steer.

Paul walked into the station, ranting to himself and waving his arms wildly. He was cursing loudly too. About the size of a small living room, the gas station was filled with a few customers, who were quietly shopping or waiting patiently to pay for their gas.

Suddenly, Paul lashed out at one girl, calling her a bitch for no apparent reason. Mary, upset but keeping her voice polite, and direct, said, "Paul, we have customers in here. You can't be talking like that."

Paul turned his eyes on her with an intensity Mary had never seen before. "He was totally different," she recalled later. "His eyes were glassy. It wasn't Paul."

"I can talk any goddamn way I want to!" Paul roared. "I own this place! You old bitch, I'm gonna kill you! I'm gonna kill you!"

Only the front counter stood between them as Paul shouted one more time, "I'm gonna kill you!"

Two customers told him to stop. Paul turned on them, calling one a bastard and chasing both of them out the door. As his father always had, Paul carried a pocketknife, and outside, he drew the three-blade knife, pulled out a blade, and flashed it at the fleeing customers.

One witness thought he heard Paul say, "I'm going to stick you, motherfucker!"

Another said Paul yelled, "You're going to die!"

More people exited the store and surrounded Paul, who started to thrust the knife at them in a stabbing motion. In the chaos that followed, one of the men ran into a tree and cut his arm. The rest backed away, and Paul stomped off down the highway, west toward Guthrie; he was ranting and pointing his finger as he talked as if arguing with someone.

Back at the station, Mary Welch had already called 9-1-1 twice. Two of the men involved in the encounter with Paul at the station jumped into their wrecker in pursuit, fearing Paul might hurt someone else. Unresponsive before when it came to Paul, this time the sheriff's office reacted, calling the Guthrie Police Department for backup.

The dispatcher reported "a man was wielding a knife and causing a disturbance at Bowman's Wrecker Service and Sinclair Station" and had cut or stabbed one of the customers, although that was later proved false. Officer Larry Wilson, on patrol alone, responded to the call. About the same age as Paul, Wilson was nonetheless five inches shorter and about forty-five pounds lighter than my brother. He spotted Paul ranting and waving his arms near the local Dairy Queen. The parking lot was full with customers' cars. It was 6:47 p.m.

Wilson pulled out his nine-millimeter Glock pistol and pointed the gun at Paul. He put up a hand as if to say "Stop." He said he couldn't tell whether Paul still had the pocketknife in his hand or not.

"Stop or I'll shoot!" Wilson commanded.

"Fuck you!" Paul was reported as screaming. "I'm going to stick that gun up your ass!"

And Paul didn't stop. He kept charging like a bull. Even for a police officer, the sight must have been frightening. Wilson, who later admitted to having been scared, kept telling Paul to stop, but the officer also steadied his aim. As my father had found all too many times, a commanding voice will not calm a schizophrenic mind.

A gun can't either. It only makes matters worse.

The officer fired.

Chapter 20

The Fight To Survive

At 6:47 p.m. Saturday, April 6, 1996, a Guthrie dispatcher reported "a disturbance/stabbing/officer-involved shooting." An ambulance was called two minutes later to a shooting at 2115 East Oklahoma. The dispatcher noted one person had already been taken to Logan Hospital in Guthrie. Paul had been shot in a confrontation with a Guthrie officer.

My brother, the former priest, was shot on the eve of the most holy day in the Catholic calendar: Easter Sunday, the day Christians celebrate Jesus's resurrection from the dead. All throughout Christendom, people would be filing into churches in the morning to hear the age-old story told again. Later this same night, in the darkness between sunset and sunrise, the first celebration of Easter would be held as Paul lay in a hospital battling for his life.

The evening call came in at home, as always, from Dad.

"Paul was shot by a police officer in Guthrie," he said. "He's being taken now to University Hospital in Oklahoma City. Wait a little, and then come down if you want."

In the aftermath of his encounter with the officer, Paul had been initially taken to Guthrie's Logan County Hospital, where he had been born during World War II, but almost immediately, doctors decided he needed to go to a top-level trauma center at one of the larger Oklahoma City hospitals. A helicopter flew Paul to University Hospital, now the OU Medical Center. In shock from the news, I did not register those details until later nor did I ask my father what had happened. My journalism career, however, had taught me that police usually aim to shoot a person in the upper half of the body, usually the chest or stomach. Surviving such a gunshot wound hinged on several factors, including how fast the victim received treatment. I knew only too well that in many cases, one shot could kill anyone.

Nan and I left our girls at home with a relative. During the twenty-three-minute drive, Nan peppered me with questions about what my father had told me. In times of family crises, she becomes the journalist, with pointed queries and then an analysis of the situation. But this time, I didn't have any answers except to say, "I don't know, but I think it's pretty serious."

We met Dad and Joy in the emergency waiting room. We learned Paul had been shot in the stomach. He was in surgery to remove the bullet—there were also bullet fragments.

Paul went into surgery at 9:00 p.m. and would remain there until 4:25 a.m. Easter Sunday, just hours before sunrise. Shortly afterward, the surgeon gave us the bad news: Paul likely would not make it. They had been unable to remove the bullet. We needed to say our good-byes. Paul was in critical condition but awake.

No one knew how long he would remain conscious.

I found my brother lying on a hospital bed with tubes attached everywhere. There was an IV fluid tube to prevent dehydration and another to provide blood flow to his undamaged vital organs. A nasogastric tube had been inserted into his nose to remove air, fluid, and blood from his stomach. An endotracheal tube was inserted into his mouth to help him breathe. He had been stripped of his clothes and covered with a white sheet. However, the man under the sheets was not the clean-shaven Paul of the past. His face was still dirty. He had long, unwashed hair and a scraggly beard.

"I'm so sorry, Paul," I said. "You can get through this. We'll be praying for you."

I put my hand on his arm. He struggled to raise his head to look at me. I could see a wild look of pain in his eyes but didn't know whether it came from the gunshot wound or from the mental illness he was fighting. Or both. For a moment I thought he was about to speak, but then he lowered his head back onto the bed, his eyes fixed on the ceiling. The hours passed slowly. The sun began to rise. Dad, Joy, our sister Marilyn, Nan, and I had all said our good-byes; the rest of the family had been notified.

Then the incredible happened: Paul began to stabilize.

On that Easter Sunday, as people celebrated the miracle of Christ's resurrection, one family received a miracle in an Oklahoma City hospital. My brother, my father's son, had lived. Ironically, no one acted as if we had just witnessed a miracle, but maybe that says more about us and our state of mind at the time than anything else. Dad and Joy took the opportunity to drive to Guthrie to see whether Paul had injured Mary Welch. My father was so ashamed about what had happened. He wanted to apologize to Mary in person on the Hight family's behalf.

On Monday, a short story about the shooting appeared in *The Daily Oklahoman*, where I worked. I had informed my supervisors that Paul had been shot, to avoid any conflicts of interest connected to the newspaper's coverage. The story reported that Paul had charged an unnamed police officer with a knife and been shot once in the chest. Despite having been shot, the story said, Paul had continued to charge the officer and knocked him to the ground. Before reading the story, we did not know what had occurred.

The next day, a longer article appeared in the *Guthrie Daily Leader* that named Officer Larry Wilson and repeated what the OSBI had said about the sequence of events. Paul had been shot but had continued to charge the officer and had knocked him down. Sheriff Doug Powell had told the *Leader* that a deputy had arrived to find Paul wrestling on the ground with the officer. The story said that despite Wilson suffering minor injuries, he and the deputy had finally restrained Paul. What the

Guthrie newspaper did not report was that the two men in the wrecker who had followed Paul from the gas station had also helped to restrain Paul. Once handcuffed, Paul was asked whether he had been shot by another officer.

"No," Paul told the officer, identified as Todd Jones. "I have lead poisoning. My stomach is hurting. Please, please . . ."

Officer Jones then helped place Paul on a backboard so he could be put into the ambulance.

On the same day the Guthrie newspaper published the story of Paul's shooting at the top of page one, a four-paragraph letter to the editor ran on the second page, next to the "Fire and Ambulance" report, right under the obituaries:

> To the Editor
> On page 25, Section A of *The Sunday Oklahoman* (March 31), it is reported that Joe Hight was promoted to assistant managing editor of *The Daily Oklahoman*.
> I was circulation manager for the *Leader* through the early seventies and hired Joe to do inserts, the mail machine and answer the complaint phone.
> He worked at this job through his senior high period. It would be the beginning of his newspaper career.
> Laurence Parker

After years of being community editor, I had been named assistant managing editor of the *Daily Oklahoman*. I was nearly thirty-eight, and the news of my promotion had had me in high spirits entering the Easter Sunday weekend. Less than a week later, the new job felt as if it had happened long ago. It would be years before I noticed the letter in the Guthrie newspaper.

However, the journalist in me had begun to ask questions about Paul's shooting and his interaction with the officer that had led up to it: How could a man who was shot in the chest or stomach continue to charge an officer? Yes, the body can absorb a great deal of energy before it is moved, but wouldn't he have at least slumped over on impact? Did the account seem out of sequence? And what had happened to the knife? Why hadn't anyone reported that Paul had been carrying a pocketknife as the Sinclair employees had stated? Yes, a pocketknife is a knife, but hardly one that would seem particularly threatening to someone with a gun, even if Paul had been flashing or waving it about earlier. Later I was told that the two men whom Paul had chased out of the service station had followed him in the wrecker and tackled Paul just after he was shot. Thus, more inconsistencies.

Then I remembered how Paul had stood—knife in hand—staring at me that day in the kitchen nearly twenty-two years before. He had not advanced on me that time, seemingly because I did not do anything to intimidate him. Could the officer have been frightened by Paul's appearance—the scraggly long hair and unkept garments? Could the officer's shouted commands have spurred Paul to further action? Could the officer have deescalated the situation by simply taking a deep breath and addressing Paul in a calm, low tone of voice? My questions were not meant to belittle what the officer had faced that night with my brother. But there were questions, I believe, that law enforcement needed to ask itself. An ill man almost died that night. No officer should have to carry such a death on his conscience, especially when there might be a way to avoid such tragic encounters.

As happens too often with stories involving people with mental illness or those living on the fringes of society, the news story from that night leaned on what the hospital and police provided without anyone having contacted any family members. According to the article in the *Daily Leader*, Officer Wilson was placed on routine administrative leave with pay after the shooting while an investigation was conducted.

"That is standard procedure," Police Chief Stephen Almon told the *Daily Leader*. "Once the OSBI completes it's [sic] investigation, we will conduct our own to make sure no policies were broken."

Assistant District Attorney Richard Smothermon told the *Leader* that his office was planning to charge Paul with assault and battery with a dangerous weapon as if the investigation were already complete and before an arrest had even been made. After several statements were taken, Smothermon needed only two days to declare that the shooting was justifiable "under the Constitution and laws of the United States and the State of Oklahoma."

Paul remained in the hospital for several days until he could be stabilized from the bullet wound and put back on his medication so he could be stabilized mentally. He was then taken to a nursing home near the state fairgrounds in Oklahoma City for rehabilitation. The family was asked to limit visitors.

I continued to ask questions, especially of my father. At the time, I had my doubts that Paul had even had a knife. I asked Dad if I could do anything else to help. "Call the district attorney's office," he said. "See about Paul's belongings and if there are any charges against him."

Dad had read the *Daily Leader* story too.

I reached the assistant district attorney and asked him about my brother's belongings, including the pocketknife that Dad said Paul might have carried on him. The assistant district attorney did not know where the pocketknife was, but he said it would be kept as evidence if found. I was polite but couldn't resist asking a few more questions, specifically about the inconsistencies in the published accounts I had seen about that night. I wondered aloud whether our family had a case against the city. I told him how the sheriff had always taken or had Paul taken to a crisis center in the past. Didn't the sheriff's office know about Paul's issues? Why hadn't the Wheatland clinic or the court responded as they had done in the past? It was no secret in Guthrie that Paul suffered from mental illness. My questions were followed by a long pause on the other end of the phone.

In the end, timing might well have saved Paul from jail.

The same day the *Leader* carried the news of Paul's shooting on page one, another story appeared below it: The OSBI was investigating Payne–Logan County District Attorney Paul Anderson for embezzlement. The same day Paul was shot, the state auditor, OSBI agents, and the state attorney general's office had raided Anderson's office. Anderson had resigned two days later. The charges claimed that the D. A. had been stealing money from the drug forfeitures account and the office's bogus check fund. I didn't know it at the time of my call, but the assistant district attorney had his own problems. When he finally broke the silence, he told me to collect Paul's belongings as soon as we wanted them.

His voice sounded tired but direct. "You don't pursue a case against the city, and we won't pursue a case against your brother."

After another pause, a shorter one. "But with one provision." Another pause. "That Paul moves out of Logan County and never returns."

I thanked him and said I needed to inform my father about the proposal. I called Dad immediately, and after running him through what had been said, I gave him the proposed deal. He didn't hesitate, "Take the deal. We'll pick up Paul's belongings tomorrow."

I made one more phone call to the D. A.'s office to say we accepted the terms. After thanking the assistant district attorney, I gave him my phone number in case he needed me for anything else. I asked him to let me know if the pocketknife was ever found. I never heard from him again. I never called his office again either. The next day, Dad picked up Paul's belongings, everything except for the missing pocketknife.

It would be years before I'd find out that after flashing the pocketknife at the gas station, Paul had tucked the small knife into the right front pocket of his jeans. After the shooting, two witnesses were asked whether they had seen Paul with the knife in his hand when he charged Officer Wilson. Both witnesses said No. Officers had found the pocketknife in his pocket when they patted him down, then placed the knife in a manila envelope and stored the envelope away.

Later, the same day the assistant district attorney ruled that the shooting was justified, Officer Wilson was interviewed again. The report filed on Wilson indicated that his firearm had been tested successfully by the OSBI, which found his nine-millimeter Glock had the proper number of rounds and that "all of the rounds were department approved ammo." An investigator then recorded the interview with the officer. Wilson, still shaken by the shooting, said he was unhappy that it had occurred. He felt he'd had no choice but to shoot Paul, because he believed his life was in danger and that "deadly force was the only recourse that he had" available to him. The officer had carried pepper spray but had not thought that would stop the charge. Earlier, Wilson had revealed that he had been thinking about firing a second shot just before Paul tackled him. In other words, if Wilson had acted on his thought, Paul might have been shot again and died at the scene.

Despite the conclusions that Paul had tried to both choke Wilson and take his gun away from him, the officer still asked, "How is Mr. Hight doing?"

That interview went into the OSBI files. We would not know until years later what Wilson had felt that night or said when questioned about it. At the time, I was still pushing for more details, but Dad had had enough. Paul had hurt his friends. Paul had embarrassed his family in the place of his birth and the community where the Hight family had lived and been respected for so many years.

A Hight would never live again in Guthrie, Oklahoma—at least in my father's lifetime.

* * * * *

The frequency at which people with mental illness come into deadly contact with law enforcement was not widely known at the time of Paul's shooting. That would not change until a 2015 *Washington Post* investigation uncovered that people with mental illness were sixteen times more likely to be shot and killed by police. In truth, about one fourth of all fatal police encounters involve someone with mental illness. The issue: a lack of training for police in how to deescalate an encounter with someone suffering from mental illness, as well as a lack of treatment for those with serious mental illness.

In Paul's case, he had been without so much: without an understanding sheriff who knew what to do with someone with mental illness. Without oversight from a mental health clinic. Without a crisis intervention plan. Without a family member who could monitor the situation closely. Without someone who could provide help without intimidation. All those withouts and more played out on that April evening in Guthrie, Oklahoma, as they continue to play out in communities across the country. Looking back, Paul's violent encounter with police seems inevitable, as inevitable as the arrival of Easter morning.

As for our Paul, we began the preparations to move him to Oklahoma City. I would visit Paul as often as I could at the nursing home where he spent several months recuperating from the bullet wound. I would take long lunch breaks from work for our visits. My early visits found him still in pain—struggling to stand and greet me. He made small steps every day. But he did make them. Eventually I was able to take him out to lunch. He was clean-shaven again and seemed to have regained the spirit that had gone missing in the heartbreak of losing Lynne.

Unknown to Paul, Dad had sold the trailer house in Guthrie and almost everything in it, as if doing so could somehow erase in people's minds what had happened that April night. As for Paul, he never asked what happened to his home or possessions. The trauma he had suffered seemed to have erased the memory.

* * * * *

On a hot August day more than three months after Paul was shot, I picked my brother up. He was still struggling physically. He winced and gave an audible gasp as he settled into the passenger seat of my car. We hadn't gone far when Paul looked over at me.

"Joe, I'm sorry for everything."

I didn't know what to say, and before I could reply, he spoke again in a soft voice.

"You know I have mental illness."

For the first time, Paul had shared with me the truth of his condition, a condition that had plagued him since his late twenties, a condition that Paul might well have not admitted to himself before. Had being shot—coming so close to death—caused this change in my brother? Maybe, maybe not. His confession, however, like a gust of Oklahoma wind, swept through the car, carrying away the pain and resentment

I had carried so long. For the first time, I felt a need to forgive Paul for scaring me with that knife all those years ago while he was off his medication. I also needed him to forgive me for being angry that he had somehow let down our family because of his mental illness, for no longer being the Catholic priest whom I had admired and aspired to be like when I was younger. He was my oldest brother, suffering from an incurable, insidious illness, who needed the love and trust of his family—my love and trust. I could give him that.

"I'm sorry this happened to you," I told him. "You will always be my big brother. I will always love you no matter what."

The awkward pause that followed recalled the first time I spoke of love to Mom over the phone so many years ago, and then, as she had, my brother replied: "I love you too."

Nothing more needed to be said.

In companionable silence, we carried on to his favorite restaurant, Mazzio's Italian Eatery and its all-you-can-eat pizza buffet and breadsticks. Paul picked at his food that day, but I remember thinking how blessed our family was. Paul had survived a police shooting. He had been given a second chance, a new beginning in Oklahoma City. He was not headed back to Griffin Memorial or worse, a county jail or state prison.

Paul looked up and gave me a big toothy grin, and my final thought before taking another bite of pizza was how fortunate I was to have my oldest brother back again. We both started to laugh. We hadn't shared such a laugh in more than two decades.

Chapter 21

A New Life

Paul never complained about the havoc the bullet wound wrought on his body or life. He never mentioned the surgical scars on his stomach and his chest—not even the incision that stretched nearly eight inches from his rib cage to lower abdomen. He never talked about the lead poisoning that might come from the bullet and fragments he still carried inside him.

Yet the stress of the shooting was written all over him. He appeared to have shrunk another half-inch in height. He had lost fifty pounds. His hearty appetite was gone, as was much of his hair. He sometimes now wore a cap to cover his receding hairline or, for dress occasions, a gray wool fedora, but he always took them off when inside. What remained of his hair was slowly turning gray, but that was probably more a factor of age than trauma. His dark blue eyes, almost hidden by the thick lenses of his tinted glasses, had dark circles under them, and they no longer shone with the confidence they had in his early priesthood. They were now the vacant eyes of a man not old but no longer young who had suffered twenty-five years of sacrifice and torment, a twenty-fifth anniversary no one would celebrate.

In that Christmas season of 1996, Paul would be turning fifty-four. He had been given a second chance, maybe his final chance to start anew, free of the trailer house in Guthrie, free of any charges from his latest trouble, free to live in Oklahoma City near family. He would never, however, be free of the voices, which seemed to grow louder and more insistent as he grew older.

As 1996 drew to a close, Paul might have found hope in a November 30 address that Pope John Paul II made to the Pontifical Council for Pastoral Assistance to Health Care Workers. The pope spoke about how Christ not only healed those who suffered from sickness in their bodies and minds but also how his compassion led him to identify with them.

> Christ took all human suffering on Himself even mental illness. Yes, even this affliction, which perhaps seems the most absurd and incomprehensible, configures the sick person to Christ and gives him a share in his redeeming passion.

Thus, the pope said, the response . . . is clear: Who soever suffers from mental illness "always" bears God's image and likeness in himself, as does every human being. In addition, whoever suffers from mental illness "always" has the inalienable right not only to be considered as an image of God and therefore as a person but also to be treated as such.

> It is everyone's duty to make an active response: our actions must show that mental illness does not create insurmountable distances, nor prevent relations of true Christian charity with those who are its victims. Indeed, it should inspire a particularly attentive attitude towards these people who are fully entitled to belong to the category of the poor to whom the kingdom of heaven belongs.

Oh, if those words of the pope could only be piped into legislatures and homes and hospitals and prisons and churches and schools the world over! The pope was begging the world to open its collective eyes and see the person, not the illness. His request recalled the efforts of missionaries who had worked with lepers in the fourteenth century and Mother Teresa's fights to abolish the caste system in India.

Back in Oklahoma City, Paul was fighting smaller battles. After spending time in a nursing home, he had been transferred to Parkview Place Apartments. Parkview was run by the Oklahoma Department of Rehabilitation Services and served as community housing for those with substance abuse or mental health issues. Paul was also receiving counseling and medication at the nonprofit Red Rock Behavioral Health Services. He always seemed happy when he was picked up from Red Rock and pensive when he was dropped off. When he finally left there, no graduation ceremony would commemorate the progress he had made as for those who overcome substance abuse. There are no graduation ceremonies for people who suffer from mental illness.

Paul seemed to be considering what his next step might be. He could have lived the life of a retiree, but was it possible that something more remained for him to do? In the fall of 1996, six months after he had been shot, Paul requested his official transcript from Cardinal Glennon College in Saint Louis. He received a student copy and another in a sealed envelope, the latter of which administrative assistant Helen M. Marx explained in a letter accompanying them:

> The reason is *official* transcripts are suppose(d) to go from institution to institution. Most institutions will accept an official copy if it comes in a school envelope that had not been opened. An official transcript bears the school seal. I hope the enclosed will help in your need. Good Luck in your endeavors. God Bless you and yours in this holiday season!

Paul never sent the sealed transcript to any college or university; instead, he opened the sealed envelope. The address listed for him on that transcript was Connections, a controversial temporary boarding house for the mentally disabled in Norman, where he had lived before relocating to Oklahoma City.

* * * * *

If Paul was going to live permanently in Oklahoma City, then he needed to find a permanent place of his own. For a person making about $7,000 annually in Social Security disability benefits and $238 a month in retirement from the state, that would not be easy. Ideally, Paul needed to find a subsidized apartment; he could furnish it thanks to the sale of the trailer house and its contents. Our sister Marilyn, easily the most outgoing of the Hight children with a soft heart for people who needed help, took the lead in helping Paul find a new home. She helped him set up a budget and counseled him on how to organize and keep his checkbook balanced, as well as the importance of maintaining a positive balance in his account. That restricted what Paul could give away to the small amount of cash or change he had in his pockets on any given day. Marilyn's plan seemed to work.

As part of the housing search, Paul received an orange folder from the Oklahoma City Housing Authority with instructions on how to apply for subsidized, or Section 8, housing. The folder contained a stapled twenty-five-page list of landlords who had one-, two-, three- and four-bedroom apartments, townhouses, or houses for rent. Some of them would have been referred to in the past as "slum landlords," opportunists who bought apartments or houses to turn them into Section 8 housing and guaranteed income. Initially, Paul had talked about the possibility of moving into Section 8 housing in Edmond, not far from where Nan and I lived, but he eventually decided that Oklahoma City would be a better choice.

At first Paul was shocked by how many addresses on the housing list turned out to be rundown apartment complexes, most of them in neighborhoods littered with abandoned homes, where residents openly peddled drugs or flashed weapons. Safety was an issue, but without a car, Paul also needed a place with easy access to the grocery store, restaurants, and convenience stores where he could get his Pepsi and cigarettes. It took a few weeks, but he found what he considered a perfect place to live: Park Manor apartments.

Paul wrote a check for $150 security deposit and paid another $195 for his first month's rent for a one-bedroom apartment at Park Manor, not far from one of the busiest intersections in the state at Northwest Sixty-Third and May Avenue and from the exclusive town of Nichols Hills, an island in the middle of north Oklahoma City and one of the richest suburbs in the country. The housing authority paid the balance of the rent, $345. The area was nice enough that at least Paul felt safe. Only two days after Christmas in 1996, he moved into Apartment No. 305, and then he and Marilyn went shopping to furnish the place. Paul needed everything from a bed to lamps to a dining table. He was starting over once again.

Paul's apartment came with a sturdy front door that had both a regular lock and a dead bolt, with a doorbell placed in the center of the door. A few of the apartments had screen doors. Paul's did not. His apartment was on the bottom floor of the complex with a front window that looked out onto the swimming pool. Paul's new community became whatever was within walking distance: French Market Mall with its Furr's Cafeteria, an IGA grocery store, a Texaco station, a Barnes and Noble bookstore, a Braum's ice cream and burger restaurant, and a small city park with basketball and tennis courts and a playground. But his favorite places to go were the IGA, Furr's, and the Texaco station. All three accepted checks from him, and with his long strides, the quarter-mile trip to the gas station was only about 475 steps.

In 1997, Paul's appetite returned, a sign that the move to Oklahoma City had been a good decision. He was still fond of all-you-can-eat buffets and often took family and guests when they visited to Furr's for its $5.62 lunch or $7.13 dinner buffets or to the nearby Hometown Buffet for its all-you-can-eat specials. He said the two restaurants reminded him of the meals that Mom fixed him when he was growing up. If Bill was in town, the brothers would cap off dinner with a movie. Paul's old friend from Guthrie, Father Hanrahan, also reentered his life. Once a month, Hanrahan would drive to the city to take Paul out for lunch— Mazzio's pizza continued to be their lunch of choice, followed by a stop at a discount smoke shop, and finally a visit to the NorthCare mental health clinic.

Hanrahan would wait while Paul had his NorthCare appointment, sometimes a few minutes, sometimes an hour. Hanrahan said he always wondered what determined the length of the sessions but felt uncomfortable asking Paul about them. The time or two he tried, Paul always quickly changed the subject, and Hanrahan could take a hint.

During this period, there were signs that Paul was feeling better about himself. He started new routines and habits, including how he dressed. His new daily attire was blue jeans and plaid shirts, topped by a black leather jacket when the weather was chilly. For holidays and special occasions, he began to favor the look of a distinguished gentleman on a budget: dark slacks, a blue or white dress shirt, a gray fedora, and in cooler weather, a classic cardigan sweater.

He also reinstated old routines. He and Mary Wheeler were back talking daily about their favorite restaurants on the phone. And he was once again calling his siblings with the latest gossip, usually about other family members but sometimes himself. That included both telling his youngest brother that women were noticing the dapper dresser he had become and sharing an occasional update on his personal life.

"I'm going on a date," he told me proudly during one conversation.
"Where to?"
"Braum's. We're going to meet there."
"Did you ask her out?"
"Nah, she asked me. I think she likes me."
"Do you like her?"
"Of course, I do, but I think she likes me more than I like her."
"So, it won't get too serious?"
"No, I can't afford for it to get too serious."

The conversation then shifted to the latest news from the rest of the family, with Paul, as usual, trying to pry information from me to be used in his other phone calls.

That March, the family traveled to Hennessey to celebrate Dad's eightieth birthday. Neither the incident at the Sinclair station, the police shooting, nor Paul's bullet wound and recovery was mentioned, as if someone had made a tape recording of 1996 and erased it. As Dad opened his presents, Paul sat beside him and watched. The grandchildren helped blow out the candles on the sheet cake that Joy had made and decorated. Dad regaled the family with stories and the destination of his and Joy's next trip.

Paul also had an announcement: "I'm going to Christ the King Church."

Father Joe Ross, who had married Nan and me, was now the pastor of Christ the King, which is located on the west side of the wealthy community of Nichols Hills. As a man of modest means, Paul would have been an exception from the typical parishioner, but he said he always felt welcomed by both pastor and congregation.

He still sat in the back during Mass, but he had gained enough confidence to join a Bible study group at the parish. He enjoyed being at the parish enough that when he couldn't get a ride, Paul would walk the almost two miles to the church.

By the end of 1997, Paul had once again built a stable life for himself, this time in Oklahoma City on a foundation of family, friends, home, and church. Despite all that he had endured, he had not given up. He was on the way to a better life.

Chapter 22

A Renewal

By the late 1990s, Pope John Paul II's Catholic charismatic renewal movement had come to Oklahoma City, reigniting Paul's enthusiasm for the universal Church. He continued his regular two-mile walks to Christ the King Catholic Church for Sunday Mass, and had added a weekly walk there for a Renewal Bible study group. More than thirty such small faith groups were ongoing at that time at the parish, Father Ross recalled. Throughout the archdiocese, many more were meeting in homes or churches.

An offspring of the Second Vatican Council, the movement had been affirmed "as the good fruits of the Renewal" by the U.S. National Conference of Catholic Bishops as early as 1968. The movement pushed the power of the Holy Spirit, the third of the Holy Trinity that includes God and his Son, lending an evangelical flavor to the universal Church. Catholic parishioners—eyes closed and arms raised high seeking power from the Holy Spirit—became a common sight at Mass. Paul was among those who felt and welcomed the enthusiasm of the Spirit, but he felt no need for such a public display. He felt it in his heart. And that was enough.

Looking back, Father Ross said he could see how the social justice issues that were part of the Renewal movement would appeal to Paul—they were not unlike his work with the poor all those years ago as a priest in Tulsa.

One of the best thing that came out of the movement could be traced to "small Catholic groups getting together. It gave a burst of energy to a lot of parishes," Ross said. "It gave voices to individuals."

For Paul, his voice came through clearly—and increasingly frequently—in his writings about God, Jesus, and the Holy Spirit and their meaning in his life. He still wrote in notebooks and notepads, but had also taken to writing note cards, sticky with cigarette residue, that he kept in a rusted tin file box. Writings and musings were commingled with phone numbers of friends, credit-card numbers, a prayer phone line, and lists, oh, so many lists.

On one white note card, he wrote in bold letters, as if he were writing a headline: "Recipe for a long good life."

Then:

1. *Keep your mouth from evil.*
2. *Keep your tongue from speaking guile.*
3. *Turn from evil.*
4. *Do good.*
5. *Seek after peace.*
6. *Pursue peace.*

Evangelical terms, such as *born again* and *being saved*, began to appear more in his writings, words commonly used in the charismatic and evangelical denominations but not traditionally in the Catholic Church.

Again, another list:

1. *Repentance: Turn from sin to virtue (for the kingdom).*
2. *Baptism & Being Born Again. Being Saved.*
3. *Persistence in Faith (Gospel).*
4. *End—Salvation.*

Then a prayer:

> *Jesus said, Be not unbelieving by believing*
> *Be a believer instead of an unbeliever.*
> *If you believe, all things are possible*
> *If you act in what you believe.*
> *Faith without works is dead, that is (an) ineffective*
> *Sad experience. God honors Faith*
> *that is acted upon no matter whether*
> *that Faith came directly or indirectly*
> *from Him. He will be the source of all*
> *ideas & words. All ideas & words*
> *are inspired by Him. People are*
> *instruments of those ideas & words.*
> *And these words are to you highly altered*
> *from that original state in God, but*
> *If you will believe and act upon them*
> *You will see results.*

Later, he wrote:

> *People are saved by calling on the name of Jesus. But first they have to hear Jesus through Preaching. (Whoever hears you, hears me.) And Preachers must be sent by whom—By God through the Christ & Her Church which is founded in Peter & the Apostles.*
>
> *Paul was called directly by Christ through a personal revelation but he submitted himself . . . Lest he be running in vain. It is entirely possible that Jesus called People to office in His Church today in a personal way & in personal revelation that those . . . should be submitted to the Church. . . .*

In 1998, Paul was a perpetually smiling, seemingly happy man. He laughed often. He spoke in ways that reflected not only his Renewal

Bible study but also his own renewed faith. The words he wrote were clear, the meaning understandable as to how he felt and what he believed. The improvement suggested that he might be returning to the state of health he had embodied before being ordained in 1968. That said, although his mental health appeared stable, Paul had begun to consider life after death, more specifically, his life after death, a transition that he believed would free him of a tormented mind and aging body.

Nearly fifty-six years old, he had lived longer than he might have expected given some of his personal health challenges; however, he had reached that age when you might think everyone around you has headed or is heading to the grave, when your peers are slowly, one by one, burying their parents. Mom was already gone, and now at eighty-one, Dad's health began to fail again. Our father had squeezed out several more years of life, years blessed with a happy marriage and travels with Joy, but now his cancer had returned, more vicious than before. Initially he decided to once again fight.

"Doctors found flecks of cancer on my lungs. You can see them in the X-rays," Dad said.

He looked devastated by the diagnosis and the audacity of the disease he had defeated once before daring to return. Cancer can destroy the physical body much like schizophrenia can destroy the mind, and the news only became more troubling for Dad. Doctors next found nonsmall cell lung carcinoma along with the return of prostate cancer. The cancer had also spread into his bones. Dad submitted to radiation and chemotherapy again. Joy became his primary caregiver. When we visited, he was usually covered in blankets and shaking uncontrollably, even in warm weather. The laughter therapy of the past wasn't going to work this time.

Before the year was out, Dad had made a decision: He would not fight the cancer anymore. Time was not on his side. Instead, he would live life to the fullest for as long as the cancer would allow him. The fact that for once, in a long time, Paul was stable and happy gave my father some relief as he neared his final days.

* * * * *

Paul did seem content, even thriving. Thanks to his parish community and medication, Paul had become almost playful, back to teasing
his family and up for revisiting hobbies he hadn't particularly enjoyed
in the past. Those included fishing with Bill and my family or celebrating an old-fashioned Fourth of July, even if our seats were so close
to the fireworks that the risk of catching fire was real. I'll never forget
how ashes, sparks, and debris rained down on us that year, until finally
everyone around us scurried off, and the Hights were the only ones who
remained. "Joe, don't you think we're too close?" Paul teased.

"What are you talking about?" I said with a deadpan look. "This is
where the *real* people see the *real* fireworks. Don't worry. They surely
wouldn't let us get this close if they thought we were in any danger."

A piece of shrapnel landed in front of me as I overheard someone
say, "I think some sparks just flew in my hair." Paul looked at me like
are you stupid?—and burst out laughing.

"Think we're too close, Joe?"

"I think we should move now!"

Paul never let me forget that night and the ribbing—"Joe, when's
the next fireworks display? Think we can get as close as we did before?"—made me feel closer to him. He felt the same way, I think. One
of the casualties of having mental illness is the loss of normalcy and the
abundance of people tiptoeing around you, worrying what to say or
not say, fretting over what to do or not do, living in fear of triggering a
relapse. Everyone ends up feeling the pressure: the person with mental
illness as well as those around that person. Few things warm a soul more
than just being there with someone, particularly a brother.

Paul had regained his spirit as well as his sense of humor. He had
developed some close relationships, including several with fellow priests,
such as Father Hanrahan. Soon other priests began to inquire about him.
Father John Petuskey, a powerful and admired force in the Oklahoma
City Archdiocese, was one. A friend of Paul's in the seminary, Petuskey
was pastor by then of Edmond's Saint John the Baptist Church, which

had become the state's largest Catholic parish. In 1998, after nine years as pastor, Petuskey had started to push to build a parish school—despite previous pastors having been vehemently opposed to the idea. Petuskey insisted a school would bring a renewed spirit to the parish. After the parish council, of which I was a member, voted to open the school in phases, one parishioner said, "Don't you realize you just destroyed our parish!" Years later, after the school opened in 1990, another person would say, "Do you know what a blessing this school has been to the parish?"

Father Petuskey began to suggest that the Church needed to help my brother more. "How is he doing?" he would ask.

"He seems to be doing well," I told him, "but he struggles at times with expenses and other needs."

"The Church should be doing more for him. Are they providing him with anything?"

"No, I don't think so."

"Well, they should. They at least should be paying his medical expenses. They at least should be paying for his glasses."

We had the same conversation several times, with Petuskey becoming ever more insistent that something must be done, that he was going to do something. And the big priest with the big heart did try. Archbishop Beltran remembered years later that Father Petuskey had pleaded with him to help Paul. "He spoke highly of Paul. All of the priests did. They had very good impressions of Paul," Beltran said. "I do remember trying to help him."

Beltran admitted, honestly, "It may have been minimal."

Eventually, Father Petuskey stopped asking about Paul. For some unknown reason, Paul had lost one of his most vocal advocates in the local Church. As the years passed, I grew more comfortable with my brother. And at church, I also became more open in telling others, including priests, that Paul was a former priest. Some shook their heads. Others smiled. More than a few, like Father Petuskey, said the local Church, the archdiocese in which Paul lived, should be doing more for Paul. My brother remained unfazed by it all, by the archdiocese's lack of concern about him, by the whispers about how a priest for life had come to no longer be a priest. His life centered on a small patch of Oklahoma City that encompassed his home and his parish. Alone in his apartment with his thoughts, he continued to write . . . and make lists:

> *If you accept God's way*
> *(Jesus) He will accept your ways*
> *as long as you do what you believe.*
> *Doing what you believe is virtue.*
> *Not acting on your belief is vice.*
> *Jesus is the way we are rooted in God, much as a plant*
> *is rooted in the ground. . . .*
> *1. Gospel is the word of God and the Power into*
> *   Salvation for all who believe.*
> *2. The word is rooted in God. . . . It takes root in you*
> *   through Faith, and you are united to God.*
> *3. . . . You cultivate the soil of faith in God by obeying*
> *   God in your life. You root out evil by refusing to reap*
> *   to what they pursue—hostility, lust, greed . . . pride,*
> *   gluttony, envy, jealously, etc.*
> *4. And the word is God and the word is Jesus.*
> *Fear, doubt, and despair are the three principal devices*
> *of the Devil (Lucifer).*
>
> *Love, Faith, Hope.*
> *1. Love is heartfelt caring that opens you to other*
> *   people and causes you to treat them right & justly . . .*
> *2. Faith is belief.*

He paused then without defining hope, as if hope were a virtue that had been denied him. Later he wrote, "God's Enterprises (are) orphans, sick people, disabled, poverty-stricken, hungry, naked (and) in prison. (And) . . . widows in their need."

Did Paul see himself in those enterprises of God as someone sick or poverty-stricken? He did not see himself as the hungry. He often talked about the weekly meals that Meals on Wheels delivered to him, which he could store in his freezer to reheat and eat later. He did not see himself as disabled, even though he was on government disability for mental illness. Maybe he was happier than most people, including his family, realized he was and did not see himself as one of God's enterprises in need of support. Certainly, no matter where Paul had landed—Tulsa, Guthrie, Norman, and now Oklahoma City—except for when his illness thrust him into the throngs of the voices, he had always been the one who found people to help, to give money, to give whatever he had. He was living his faith in the world, just as Vatican II had asked Catholics to do—could it be that it never occurred to him that he might warrant a little grace?

Paul's writings reveal that he believed helping others included listening, clarifying, comforting, adoring his Lord, and emphasizing faith through talking about what he called "my hard experience." He defined helping others as "practical assistance" and "actual love." He wrote about the percentages of money that should go to a ministry, to feed the hungry, to help the Church. And despite the good he continued to do, one sentence defined his feeling about what his life had become:

I missed my true vocation which was to help people.

He never realized that he was helping people through his own life, through the example of his simple, honest life. Paul had regained faith and purpose in Oklahoma City. However, his faith would be severely tested in what transpired the next year, the last year of the millennium, the year of hell.

Chapter 23

The Year from Hell

Death stalked my family in 1999. Death stalked Oklahoma. Death stalked the world. And death may have started to stalk Paul, although no one realized it at the time. The words sound dramatic as I write them, but I assure you that is exactly how I felt that year. I hated 1999—hated the last year of the millennium with a passion, and not because of some ridiculous trumped-up fear over the Y2K computer bug or crazy talk about the end of times. I hated 1999 for the senseless, painful loss of life that it would bring.

On Monday, May 3, 1999, a massive killer tornado barreled into Oklahoma, only a little more than four years after the Oklahoma City bombing. The community was still recovering from the worst domestic terrorist act in the country's history, when God's wrath, as some, including my brother Paul, called cyclones, descended on the Oklahoma City metro like the dust clouds that had enveloped the state during the Dust Bowl. Only this black cloud left nothing behind—it stripped the landscape bare. Record winds of more than three hundred miles per hour generated multiple tornadoes, including some of the strongest ever recorded. The tornadoes mowed over what they didn't toss or suck into the heavens: cars, houses, and lives. The largest tornado, more than a mile wide, stayed on the ground for an unbelievable hour and a half. Forty-six people died, thirty-six alone in the suburb of Moore, south of Oklahoma City.

Later, Rick Mitchell, then chief meteorologist at KOCO-TV in Oklahoma City, would observe, "We really didn't take tornadoes seriously until 1999. Until then, it was like, 'We get tornadoes here. It's Oklahoma, but it's no big deal.' The May 3 tornado outbreak: It changed people's perceptions." Mitchell was among the meteorologists, along with local weather forecasting legend Gary England, credited with saving lives that day. More than a month later, our newspaper was still logging long hours to provide the day-to-day coverage the community needed as it struggled to recover.

In one of the year's few bright spots, just before my forty-first birthday, I was named one of two managing editors at *The Daily Oklahoman*. I could see the responsibilities that would come with the promotion; but I was blind to the wave of loss headed our way.

That month, Nan and I watched my brother-in-law, Martin, die from cancer, a disease that had changed him from a skeptical, almost cynical, educator into a warm, caring man who only wanted to be with his family. He had recently converted to Catholicism, and Paul had rejoiced at the news. In July, two of my wife's cousins, affectionately called Uncle Jules and Aunt Xenia, died within a week of each other. I wrote their obituaries and spoke at both services. Virginia Fox Crumb, better known as Nan's Aunt Dudie, died in October, leaving behind a fifty-year-old daughter growing weaker from lymphoma. Beth Ann Knight would follow her mom in less than four years, as I became accustomed to writing death notices for family.

Cancer was also consuming my father. He had made it to the age of eighty-two, but his chances of seeing the new century were poor. When we visited Joy and Dad in Hennessey, I had taken to reminiscing with him about the past and about my childhood—silly family stories at the time but that now meant so much. I reminded him how the worst seat in the family car was right behind him because with the window open, an Oklahoma wind was certain to blow some of his Copenhagen chewing tobacco right in the occupant's face. Oftentimes, since I was the youngest, that seat was mine. Teasingly, I accused him of being ornery enough to have done it intentionally. I revisited one of his and Uncle Lee's classic bull-shoots about how I was born the biggest baby known to mankind and then recapped some of his best Sunday lectures from our childhood. I talked about what he had taught us—the lessons we would not only never forget but would also work to instill in our own children in future years.

Dad would listen as I remembered, wincing occasionally in pain. Every now and then, he would manage a tight little smile, but never the hearty laugh of his storytelling days that I so wanted to hear again. Occasionally, Paul came with us, and he was surprisingly jolly company, but Dad didn't seem to notice that his oldest son, once plagued by voices and anxiety, was stable and doing well on his own. Instead, Dad would talk about what needed to be done after he died, and as always, his requests were direct.

"You'll have to watch over Paul more. You're the trustee over that trust. Use it if you have to."

"Yes, I know. Don't worry."

"One other thing: After I'm gone, don't ever quit seeing Joy. She took care of me when I was sick. I love her. Promise me."

"I promise, Daddy," I said. "She's the only grandma my children have ever known. She will always be their grandma. I always will remain close to her."

Eventually the cancer worsened, and Dad moved into Saint Mary's Regional Medical Center in Enid. To relieve Joy, my sister Susan, who lived in Wichita, Kansas, would drive in to sit with Dad when she could. I made the drive almost every evening after work. I knew the end was near, and I wanted, no, needed, to spend as much time as possible with my father. Late at night, I would hear Dad mumbling about a barn, a shed, and a tank. The murmurs were unintelligible, and they always seemed to upset him. One night, the mumbling woke him, and I decided to ask him about them.

243

"Tell me about the barn, Daddy."

He didn't reply.

"Why do you need to get to the tank?" I asked.

He didn't reply.

"I don't understand, Daddy. Why do you keep talking about the barn and the tank?"

He looked at me with sad eyes but was asleep before I could ask again. Later in the night, the mumbling started again, only this time, he seemed to be urgently trying to say something to me.

"Daddy, what can I do? Please tell me."

"The barn and tank, I have to go there now!"

"I don't understand. Why do you have to go there?"

His words faded away to a low murmur. Nearly fifty-one years after Linda's death, my father's mutterings seemed to be a final effort to change the outcome of that tragic day. I knew losing Linda had devastated my parents, as such a loss would any mother or father, but I realized I had no idea how close to the surface the horror still ran for my father, the horror of not getting to the water tank soon enough to save her. More than half a century later, nearly on his deathbed, her death was the one that haunted him.

On Sunday, November 14, 1999, I drove to the care center in Hennessey where Dad had been placed as he became increasingly unresponsive. His body had no more fight left. The pastor of Saint Joseph's, Father Mark Mason, was there giving him last rites. I, however, still had something I needed to say to Dad, although I could barely choke out the words.

"I love you, Daddy. Thank you for being my dad."

There was nothing more to do or say. The call from Joy came less than two hours later, shortly after I had returned to Edmond.

"Joe," she said, "Wilber just died."

I wrote my father's obituary too.

Unknown to us, Uncle Lee, my father's storytelling cohort, had also died in Oregon. The Hight brothers had died within three days of each other. Uncle Lee at the age of ninety-two and my father, ten years younger. We buried my father next to Mom and Linda. A white marble marker with a Latin cross chiseled above his name read:

MT SGT US MARINE CORPS WORLD WAR II.

* * * * *

In the aftermath of Dad's death, Paul remained steadfastly optimistic and the rock of the family. As he had when our mother died, he simply maintained that our father was in a better place. "He is in heaven. He is with Mama again," Paul repeatedly assured me. Unlike I had with my mother, I accepted Paul's reasoning more this time. Not until years later would I learn that Paul had had his own personal issues and problems in 1999. One incident was immortalized on a yellowed Oklahoma City Police Department citizen's assistance form:

> To better provide you with information concerning your case with the Oklahoma City Police Department, the following information is provided.

The card showed the name of a police office, the nature of the crime (a robbery with a firearm, a case number, and the date). On the back, the phone number for the department's investigations bureau had been circled. A police report filed on March 3, 1999, gave the reason: While walking the quarter-mile from the Texaco station back to his apartment at 4:30 a.m. that Wednesday, a pickup with three people inside, had suddenly pulled up beside Paul and stopped. "Motherfucker, give us your money!" the driver yelled, as one of the passengers jumped out of the truck and pulled a gun on Paul. Sticking the gun in Paul's side, the man reached into Paul's right front pants pocket and took his wallet. He asked only one question. "Do you have any gold?"

"No," Paul said, "I just have brass."

The man jumped back in the car, and the truck drove away with its lights off. Paul walked on home. Afterward, Paul told police that he could identify the man with the gun, but no one was ever arrested—possibly no one even followed up. Paul lost his wallet, his driver's license, debit and ATM cards, and a one-dollar bill. The irony was that if they had only asked, Paul would have given them the money.

Unknown to our family, in August a manager at the nearby IGA that Paul frequented made a call to police about a $72.48 check a man had presented to one of the cashiers. The cashier had recognized the name on the check as a regular customer, Paul Hight. When asked about it, the man told the cashier that Paul was "home sick and wants me to get him some groceries . . . I have his driver's license." The cashier recognized Paul's face on the driver's license and took the check. Later that same day, Paul came in to write a check for cash.

"I thought you were sick," the cashier said, and she proceeded to tell Paul about the check she had taken from the man she did not know.

When the police asked, Paul explained that a homeless man had come to his door the previous week and asked for a place to stay. Paul had taken the man in, but he did not know the man was using his checkbook and had his driver's license. The police had a good description of the culprit, but the case was never pursued. Paul didn't want to prosecute. He thought the man needed the groceries and money more than he did.

Through that Christmas and into the New Year, despite attending family gatherings and seeing his siblings, Paul never mentioned either incident. We'll never know why. We could only hope 2000 would be a better year. For Paul. For all of us.

Chapter 24

The Jolly Patriarch

Paul entered the new millennium as the new patriarch of the Hight family, a replacement for the father we had lost in the hell that was 1999. Our oldest brother assumed the role naturally, especially as it pertained to me, his youngest brother. His long ritual of calling his siblings to gather their news and then share it with everyone else served him well in his new position in the family. I found myself to turn to Paul for advice—which often, no matter the situation, was to remain optimistic.

"God will take care of you," he would say.

That Christmas, Paul gave me a rustic-style, battery-operated plastic clock, knowing I was something of a clock collector. Journalists are always on deadlines and watching the clock because of it, so clocks, watches, and just about anything else that can tell time hold a disproportionate importance in their lives. The clock immediately went on my desk at *The Oklahoman*. Christmas and birthday gifts from Paul were always chosen with much thought and often had a spiritual overtone. One Christmas, he gave Nan and me a copy of the poem "Footprints," nicely matted and framed. In allegorical prose, a person dreams of walking on the beach with God only to ask why in the lowest, saddest times of his life, God had left him to walk alone—leaving one, not two sets of footprints in the sand.

> The Lord replied, My precious, precious child, I love you and would never leave you. During your times of trial and suffering, when you saw only one set of footprints, it was then that I carried you.

I have found a place for that gift from my brother in every home that we have owned since. The poem reminds me of all the hardship and lonely trials Paul had endured in his life and what, in the aftermath of our father's death, he was trying to take on of mine and my family's.

By the end of his first year as the Hight family patriarch, he was thriving, buoyed in part by a sense of newfound respect. By December 2000, having turned fifty-seven, he was as joyful as I had ever seen him. He had regained most of his weight. He had replaced all that he had lost in the previous year's robbery. He approached daily life with a smile, a hearty laugh, and an exuberance usually reserved for the young. He was even laughing in his new photo on his driver's license. Once averse to human touch, Paul now didn't hesitate to accept a friendly hug from a family member or friend.

He was still making about the same in Social Security disability, along with the small retirement check. His subsidized rent was $154, and thanks to my sister's help, he was keeping to a budget. He lived frugally but was able to pay his bills and have enough left for the meal specials at Furr's Cafeteria.

A believer in the importance of tithing, a practice that was gaining favor in Catholic parishes, he gave five to ten dollars a week to his parish as well as other good causes. He was still walking most places but now occasionally opted for a bus or cab to attend church or go elsewhere if he was in a hurry. His friend Father Hanrahan still stopped by once a month to take him to the NorthCare clinic for medication management and his monthly shot of the antipsychotic Haloperidol, or

Haldol. NorthCare charged $15 for the Haldol shot and $86 to $100 for the medication management, the latter of which was designed to ensure that the right medicines and dosages were being taken. Of that cost, Paul was responsible for $3 for the shot and as much as $22 to $24 for the medication management. His appointments were usually at 11:00 a.m. with a doctor or nurse, so the two old friends had time to visit the smoke shop and Mazzio's afterward. Paul was back to enjoying breadsticks again.

With Paul doing so well, we could take a break, if only temporarily. Worrying about a family member with mental illness can be exhausting, wondering whether the next phone call will break the calm, trying to refrain from prying or pouncing on any odd change in behavior.

Those odd changes had already started to occur with Paul. We just hadn't noticed yet. One was that whenever anyone came to take him out for any reason—lunch, dinner, or an outing, Paul now insisted on meeting them outside, not at his front door. At first I shrugged it off. Knowing Paul wasn't a particularly good housekeeper, I assumed he hadn't tidied up and was embarrassed about the mess. But photos would later reveal that Paul's new reluctance to have anyone in his apartment might have stemmed from his purchase of a citizens band radio and a police scanner. He was not talking to anyone on the devices but using them to listen in on police and other transmissions.

As the year unfolded, Paul continued his spontaneous writings, including his analysis of the Bible and all that had happened to him the previous year. The small faith group meetings had ended, but Paul seemed to have individually carried on their work. In one writing, he wrote that salvation and the kingdom of God would be obtained "by keeping the commandments":

> *1.? Thou shalt not steal. 2. Thou shalt not bear false witness. 3. Thou shalt not kill. 4. Thou shalt not covet other's things. 5. Thou shalt not commit adultery. B. By giving to the poor and following Christ. C. By forgiveness of sin when you lose it.*

When you lose it was an odd phrase, but could have meant that he thought others had lost their way by committing a sin. Or he had lost his way when the voices took over. He privately admitted to a few friends that the voices were getting stronger as he aged. The medication was not working as well as it had.

Then he wrote something that might have been personal to him. He capitalized certain words for emphasis.

> *The Penalty of sin is poverty, sickness and death. Jesus took the Penalty upon Himself? Jesus became poor that we might be rich. Jesus took our infirm(ities) upon Himself that we might be healed. By his sacrifice we are healed. God sent His only begotten Son so that All who believe in Him might not Perish but have eternal life. Salvation is not a matter of works, but a matter of Faith, Belief in the Lord Jesus. Jesus clothes us with His righteous. Jesus is Lord. The Law has all been Fulfilled by Jesus and in Jesus.*

Was he talking about his own life? Was he talking about others who had hurt him? Had he begun to think his *eternal life* was approaching? Paul had to know that his health, both physically and mentally, was beginning to falter and that the gunshot wound had shortened his life. Other changes hinted that Paul might again be on the decline. Once again, he was getting up at all hours of the night to walk. Maybe his renewed late-night trips to the Texaco station had prompted him to buy the scanner so he could monitor any possible dangerous activity before venturing outside alone. Since Paul had once been mugged so close to home, one could understand what might lead him to do so. Still, Paul remained his jolly, pleasant self when around his family. In later years, I would wonder if that had been the real Paul or an act he maintained to keep him from being committed to another mental hospital.

At the beginning of 2000, we received the news that our father would be inducted posthumously into the Guthrie Sports Hall of Fame in his old hometown. I had been asked to speak on our father's behalf.

Joy, Paul, and other family members attended the induction, and Paul positioned himself directly in front of the podium where I would speak.

On accepting the award on behalf of the family, I noticed Paul staring intently as I gave this short speech:

> On behalf of my family, I want to say how honored and touched we are in receiving this award for my father. But in accepting it, I want to tell you about Wilber Hight. First and foremost, he was a tough man, a survivor.
>
> He survived being poor during the Dust Bowl days of Oklahoma and the Great Depression.
>
> He survived World War II. The Japanese suicide missions at Guadalcanal in the Pacific. Being stranded off the waters of an island in which the Japanese were eating anything they could find, including prisoners. Malaria.
>
> He survived the tragic drowning of his second child, a daughter named Linda.
>
> He survived—probably through faith—the trials and tribulations of raising his six other children. He would sit them all on the couch after church on Sundays and proclaim in dramatic form that they were all born to be leaders.
>
> He survived through the hell of cancer, once beating it when he was sixty-five.
>
> And he survived many other things.
>
> How did he survive?
>
> By being 'rough as a cob,' he would say.

I looked out onto the audience and noticed Paul smiling and nodding. He seemed to be taking in my every word.

> Although he died last November at age eighty-two, he left a legacy—his second wife, Joy, his children, his

grandchildren and his 'adopted' children—many of whom are here this evening. And, all of his children have done well in life. They all graduated from college, and many worked toward or have advanced degrees. So his ultimate achievement goes beyond those days on the football field. It's the achievement of not only surviving as a father but achieving as one too.

When I finally finished, I didn't listen for the applause. Instead, I looked for Paul. My oldest brother, now our family's patriarch, was grinning broadly, pleased and proud, it seemed.

* * * * *

The days and months passed quickly that year, as often happens when you have children, a demanding job, and other obligations. I had become involved in the founding of the Dart Center for Journalism and Trauma, now based at Columbia University and dedicated to ethical coverage of violence and tragedy, and I was traveling more as a result. Paul and I still talked on the phone once or twice a week. He remained a great listener, always eager to hear about my latest trip, about the girls, about Nan. He wasn't shy about offering advice or assuring me that God was watching over me. As a family, we saw him as often as we could, but looking back, it doesn't seem enough.

"Joe, Daddy and Mama are proud of you." Paul always spoke in the present tense when talking about our parents. To him, they were still with us. As for me, I believed their spirits were within us.

"Well, they are proud of you too," I said.

"Well," he said in a wry tone, "I don't know about that."

What I didn't realize, what no one seemed to realize—not Father Hanrahan, not the doctors at the clinic, not Father Ross, not the people at church—was that the voices were once again speaking loud and adamant in Paul's mind. He had taken to sitting in his chair and pounding his head against the wall to eject them. Sometimes he slammed his head so hard that he left bloodstains on the wall. He began to do the same while sitting up in bed at night, if he went to bed at all. Our father's death had affected Paul more than any of us knew. His grieving, kept mainly from the family, had served to intensify the emotions he felt, and it had also intensified the voices in his mind that sought to gain a permanent grip on him. Paul continued to present a happy, stable demeanor, but inside, he was being tormented again.

The evidence of Paul's secret decline was obvious only in his writings from 2000. They became erratic. The numbers. The repeated names. The mixture of spiritual feelings with earthly emotions. All hidden in his apartment from anyone who could help him. In an envelope marked "Open Dec. 27, 2003," a folded piece of notepad paper lists several names, ending with a notation that Paul becomes a supervisor of AT&T on December 26, 2000, and manager of H&R Block by fall 2005 "provided I go to school now." Another note card read: "Paul W. Hight identity card" on the outside and "12:44 am 2050. I'm due A 63rd & May Texaco to register my name. Eric Peterson." But the most telling writing came on a Trinity Broadcasting Network New Birth Certificate. A majestic logo of a golden crown and a crest of the Holy Spirit and the cross topped the certificate, but on the left side of the logo, Paul had written "You Big Hypocrite. You Liar" and on the other side, "Final Name: Wilber Eugene Joseph Hight." Underneath the logo, the word "motherfucker" had been written, the slur that had been hurled at him during the armed robbery in 1999.

The certificate was covered in random names: Buddy Ebsen, the patriarch on the 1960s sitcom *The Beverly Hillbillies*; Michael Carson, possibly half of the San Francisco Witch Killers of the 1970s; and Johnnie Walker Red, a brand of classic Scotch whiskey. Theirs and others' covered both sides of the certificate in no discernible pattern. The certificate began:

> This is to acknowledge that [blank] has accepted Jesus Christ as Lord and Savior and having confessed and been forgiven of sins by the blood of Christ is reborn by the spirit of God into the body of Christ.

Paul had filled in the blank, "Paul Wilber Polycarp Hight." Polycarp was a second-century Christian bishop who was burned at the stake by the Romans. Some accounts claimed that when the fire did not consume him, he was stabbed to death. In other accounts, the fire burning Polycarp smelled like bread baking. As for why Paul listed the name of this martyr as his own, none of his writings say.

Father Hanrahan had noticed that Paul's visits at NorthCare seemed to be getting shorter and shorter. But no one in the family was notified that anything was wrong. According to a Medicare summary notice, Paul received a Haldol shot on October 31, 2000.

On November 3, when the University of Central Oklahoma honored me as a Distinguished Former Student, Paul was once again sitting right in front of the podium so that I could see him clearly when I gave my speech. This speech was lighthearted, and Paul laughed loudly at each small joke. Eventually I noticed that even when I wasn't joking, Paul was laughing.

He was the first to hug me after the official photo was taken. He had indeed almost transitioned into a father figure for me, so I was touched when after the hug he said, "We're very proud of you, Joe."

I knew he meant it. But when I looked directly into his eyes, they didn't seem right. With a crack in my voice, I asked, "Is everything okay, Paul?"

"Yes, it is, Joe! Perfectly fine!" Paul exclaimed, and then he chuckled and said, "I loved your speech. It made me laugh!"

In that moment, I feared Paul was far from perfectly fine, but in the excitement of the evening, my concerns were not pursued and were soon forgotten. Paul's laughter was a masquerade. He knew that being belligerent could cause issues, possibly even recommitment to an institution or, worse, a call to the police. He was trying to hold onto his independence, trying to laugh through the torment in his mind that was becoming increasingly persistent and serious.

By Thanksgiving, when the family gathered at our home in Edmond for the holiday, Paul was cheerful but taking more breaks to smoke outside. After dinner, he volunteered to help Marilyn with the dishes, and as he chatted with his youngest sister while they washed the plates and saucers, Paul announced, "I'll be the next one to go."

More than a year had passed since Dad's death. None of us knew that Father Hanrahan had become ill and was no longer visiting Paul, which meant no one had been taking Paul for his monthly shot. Even as Paul revealed to Marilyn his fear that he would be the next Hight to die, he did not mention any of the changes in his routine.

The situation shows the fragility of caring for an independent adult with mental illness: You want to encourage independence and self-reliance, especially when the person is doing well. Think how insulted most of us would be if someone was always second-guessing our decisions. But if Paul had provided an emergency contact to NorthCare, a person to call if he quit showing up for appointments or seemed to be doing poorly, the clinic had not used it. And without such considerations or safeguards, Paul and others with mental illness face situations that can quickly turn tragic or even deadly.

Chapter 25

The Final Days

Paul sat at the table amid the clutter of paper, matchsticks, and dirty glasses, making a budget for Christmas gifts. Behind him, bloodstains caked the wall; near his feet, burn marks stained the brown carpet. Tattered receipts were scattered everywhere. He had a little more than two hundred dollars in the bank to cover both his December bills and his Christmas list. He had not received his monthly shot in November, so his mind was becoming as jumbled a mess as his house. As the old voices grew louder and more strident, new voices joined the chorus pounding in his head. No one knew of the return of the voices except for Paul.

He struggled to concentrate on the task at hand: prioritizing the money he had over bills and gifts for the family. No. 1 on the list: "Rent. Christmas for kids. Education. Food. Cigarettes. Electrict. [sic]," he wrote. He must have then remembered his nieces' upcoming birthdays, one of whom was also his goddaughter, because he listed for No. 2: "Birthdays Rebecca and Elyse. Loans. Runs to the station. Phone. Tithe & offering on credit card." He had no priorities under No. 3, but No. 4 included dry cleaning. The latter probably didn't rate any higher spot on the list because Paul was not changing his clothes or bathing very often.

The rest of the paper held a scattershot of numbers, more numbers, and even more numbers that didn't make any sense. He appeared to be struggling to find a balance among what he wanted, what he had to do, and what would settle his mind and quiet the voices. But the voices were relentless. They told him what he needed was more money, which seemed to have sent Paul scrambling for any slip of paper he could find on which he wrote imaginary monetary windfalls. One said he would be receiving $6 billion in his bank account. Grantland Rice would pay him five dollars an hour, twenty-four hours a day in five days. Fifty "billion, trillion dollars per millennium" was coming in for food, and "60 billion trillion" was expected soon for cigarettes. His numbers estimated an immediate influx of "280,000 dollars per month." The numbers were blurred by coffee stains and punctuated by cigarette burns.

For someone who had so little money, Paul's clouded mind was now consumed with it. The man who had always given away money to anyone who asked was now on a strained budget. Greed was not behind the numbers scattered throughout his apartment, but desire. Paul wanted to have enough money to buy Christmas presents for all his nieces and nephews and for his family—and to fulfill his obligations to his landlord, the Church, and the poor. Only those who have sat in his place at Christmastime, with all the expectations the holiday brings, could understand the financial pressure he was under to accomplish all that.

On the table, a newsletter announced the Christ the King Catholic Church holiday schedule. Paul planned to attend the Advent Penance Rite on December 17. He had already given much thought to what was "essential to the abundant life." On a page torn from a green notepad, he had begun to write:

1. Health, spiritual . . . physical.
2. Prosperity material.
3. Spiritual prosperity.
4. Freedom to all & (to) find a future in God and others.

The numbers 5 to 10 all mention freedom.
The rest of the page is blank.

The healthy Paul might well have been surprised that material prosperity had trumped spiritual prosperity on his list—if he had not had his other concerns on his mind and coming through the police scanner.

During the previous ninety days, three people had been shot and killed by Oklahoma City police officers. That brought the total to ten police-involved shootings for the year. Local media had been comparing the frequency to other cities in the region, and Oklahoma City had not fared well. One fatal shooting in the previous seventeen months in the entire Dallas/Fort Worth, Texas, area. One fatal shooting of three police-involved shootings in Tulsa, on the other side of the state. The latest local shooting had been Friday morning, December 1, when forty-three-year-old Deborah Conley Gregory was seen carrying a knife as she walked along an Oklahoma City street. Two officers, with weapons drawn, followed the woman for several blocks and then confronted her and ordered her to drop the knife. When instead of doing what they asked the woman tried to cross a street toward a school, they started to fire. Gregory died of a bullet wound to the stomach, and the officers were cleared quickly by the Oklahoma County district attorney's office.

Normally the incident might have gone unnoticed, but with the media spotlighting the rise in police shootings, the Oklahoma City Police Department was becoming defensive. "When you use any type of force you are taught to use that force until that threat is no longer there," Sergeant Cris Cunningham told KOCO-TV on December 6. "If someone is coming at you with a knife, you're not going to shoot the knife out of their hands."

The shooting soon was overshadowed, as so many matters are in Oklahoma, by the weather. The KOCO forecast called for snow or an ice storm or both by early the next week. By Friday, the possibility of a winter storm blanketed the airwaves. In his apartment, Paul picked up references to the impending storm but continued to work on his Christmas list. The possibility of snow or ice leaving him homebound didn't worry him. He had enough food. Mobile Meals had made another delivery, and he had stored the meals in the freezer. Furr's was nearby, and there were always the snacks at the Texaco station.

He squinted to bring the names and numbers into focus. He had either lost or broken his big, thick-lensed glasses. The voices were telling him that he didn't need them anyway. Lately, he had been losing a lot of things, including his Social Security card. A replacement had just arrived in the mail. But as he squinted again to see what he was writing—and most likely failed, he decided to make a phone call.

I answered and heard, "Joe . . . ," followed by a long pause. I recognized my brother's voice.

"Paul, are you okay?"

"Yes, perfectly fine," he said, "but I've lost my glasses and need to get some new ones. Do you know where I could go?"

"You could go to my eye doctor," I said. "We'll see if we can make an appointment before the storm."

"Okay, one more thing: I also need to get my monthly shot. Could you or Nan take me?"

"Well, yes, I think Nan could. I'll ask. Hey, would you want to have lunch? We could go to Earl's barbecue on Western."

"Yeah, that would be great!" He sounded more enthusiastic than when he had begun the call. "But we need to go before the storm. Could we go on Monday?"

"I'll check."

Everything fell into place: Nan was available. Paul could get his shot in the morning and then see the eye doctor in the afternoon. We could go to Earl's Rib Palace in between for lunch.

The sad truth is that a person can hold more than one thought at the same time—and they needn't all be happy ones. While Paul was expressing enthusiasm about future doings to me, possibly because he didn't want me to worry about him, he was expressing doubts about his life to others. Jerry Lindsley, a longtime friend of Paul's from Guthrie, was one of the people in whom Paul confided, and he had picked up a concerning refrain from my brother.

"You can't psychoanalyze," Lindsley said, "but [Paul] made a remark to me that he was tired of living. Tired of the way he was living. Tired of taking medication."

Neither his friend nor Paul's writings indicated that he felt death was imminent. Paul appeared to think his death was still years away. On one piece of paper, he had written the time, "12:30 Feb. 21, 2001." By that weekend, he might have made a prediction on one of his note cards in that rusted green box:

D Day 11:15 July 12, 2005.
Death 11:32:25 March 26, 2005.

He needed a shot of medication quickly. Nothing was making sense anymore. He was feeling nervous as he waited for Nan to pick him up that Monday, which might have been because of the upcoming storm. Even though the high was not expected to top 25 degrees Fahrenheit that day, Paul was up early, walking the nearly five hundred steps to and from the Texaco station in the frigid cold. Together, Nan and I spent nearly five hours with my brother that day, but he still managed thirteen trips to the nearby gas station to buy drinks or refills for his Pepsi.

Snow was expected later that evening. Rain and snow were expected Tuesday. Snow and a thunderstorm were expected on Thursday. Temperatures each night would be in the teens, and wind chills would be below zero. Schools, churches, businesses, and just about anything else that could do so would close for at least part of the week. The exceptions would be the media, law enforcement, hospitals and ambulances, state emergency transportation workers, and maybe some convenience stores, gas stations, and fast-food joints. Most people took it in stride—schoolchildren welcomed a potential snow day, grownups a cozy day at home to watch movies or read. However, for people who suffer from paranoid schizophrenia, icy weather, along with the lack of sunshine that comes with it, can cause increased anxiety and anger because it interrupts routines that people use to cope with their illness.

Paul was already paranoid, but he now suspected someone, perhaps someone he'd befriended in his apartment complex or taken in, of stealing his Social Security number and possibly his disability payments. And he might well have been correct. Social Security Administration records showed his last benefit as going to a 44210 zip code in Summit County, Ohio, with the address of his last residence being in Duncan, Oklahoma. Paul had never lived in or likely visited either place.

Despite these growing concerns, Paul expressed no such worries when Nan picked him up for his eleven o'clock appointment at NorthCare, despite having jotted down on one of his notes a phone number, followed by "[Frank Sabovich] Assassin." Instead, he had done his best to make himself presentable, although his chin was bleeding slightly as if he had nicked himself shaving.

He and Nan caught up during the car ride over, with Paul excited about the rest of the activities planned for the day, especially going for ribs for lunch. He spent fifteen minutes at NorthCare, with Medicare records showing he received the shot as planned but no "medication management" as before. That omission had nothing to do with his tight budget; he had already "met the Plan B deductible for 2000," so ability to pay wasn't an issue. No one seems to have asked why he had not received a shot in November.

Before I left for work to meet them at the rib place for lunch, Nan called me to say Paul seemed off, but he was excited about lunch and seeing me. I arrived to find Paul with a wild look in his eyes but cheerful. I had seen Paul like this before and knew that it meant he was off his medication—his mood swung from mischievous to distant, from engaged to distracted, with a laugh that recalled Vincent Price's in Michael Jackson's *Thriller* video. Very likely, the morning shot had not yet had time to compensate for the November shot he had missed, but that also might have been expecting too much from one shot. As we hugged, I smelled the stench of cigarettes. If possible, the smell was stronger than usual.

As we talked during lunch, I noticed Paul looking past me. He would lose focus, smile broadly, and then refocus on our conversation. He burst out once in loud laughter, and then, seeing my puzzled expression, quickly dismissed it, saying, "Oh, it's nothing." I couldn't help but wonder if he was trying to listen not only to me but also to the voices. Still, I was optimistic that the morning's medication would kick in soon and stabilize Paul. The shot would bring my jovial brother back. I didn't know then that without other medication, the shot could take as long as six days to take effect.

As we hugged good-bye, I reminded Paul that the snowstorm was expected soon and to stay safe and warm inside. He nodded and gave a little chuckle as he walked to Nan's vehicle. I waved good-bye, saying "I love you." Paul stopped and flashed me a broad, toothy grin as I promised I would see him after the storm. He was in such high spirits, I felt assured the medication had started to work. Nan would get him to the optometrist, and he would soon get new glasses.

Everything would be okay.

* * * * *

The winter storm hit hard, spreading snow and ice over the state like a slick frosting. Schools closed on Tuesday. Ice sculptures formed at nearby lakes. Temperatures rose to only 17 degrees Fahrenheit the next day, dropping to 10 degrees Fahrenheit that night. The combination of snow topped with ice made it impossible to walk outside safely. Paul still tried. He made three trips to the Texaco station that Tuesday. The scanner was crackling—first responders were responding to calls from all over the city. The citizens band radio was chirping.

As for my brother, he was holed up indoors, writing, "Paul Wilber Polycarp Hight" over and over. He jotted down the names of different professions. He wrote Dad's name. He wrote, "Slavery is condemned. Paul W. Hight Pres. Finished & Fired Yahweh." He might also have been banging his head on the wall again. His condition worsened the next day. The temperature was still below freezing, and any melted snow had refrozen. Getting around outside was still treacherous, but that didn't stop Paul. He had run out of Pepsi and was twitching from a lack of caffeine. In his mind, I'm sure he thought he had no choice but to make a run to the gas station.

Paul talked loudly to the voices as he walked. He was back to batting away at them too. Inside the Texaco station, he went to pour a fountain drink, but something caused him to groan so loudly in frustration that the few other customers in the store turned and stared at him. He yelled at the clerk about his perceived issues, paid his money, and stormed out of the store. Back in his apartment, an all too familiar routine began to play out: Paul started to scream, throw chairs around the room, and punch at the demons inside his head. He couldn't run away into the frigid night, but he opened his front door to the cold, where he stood, staring into the night. He had on a coat, pants, and sandals, neighbors would report later, but no shirt. He showed no emotion.

This continued for several days.

"Paul, are you okay?" asked his neighbor Isabel as she passed by on her way to close the laundry.

Paul nodded but said nothing else.

The cold weather continued. Snow still covered the ground. The streets retained an icy glaze. Most people remained inside or adjusted their routine to be outside as little as possible. Cooped up in his apartment, Paul became more agitated and paranoid. By the next day, the sunshine had returned, glistening so brightly against the snow that it was difficult to look outside without squinting.

Paul's shot, however, still wasn't working, and the voices had begun to taunt him. He became convinced that his next-door neighbors were part of the conspiracy against him. He started to bang on the walls. He walked to the Texaco station two more times. He called no one. No one thought to call him. The snow and ice had taken everyone's focus away, leaving a fifty-something man to fight his demons alone.

That evening as the paranoia intensified, Paul stepped outside and took two short steps to Apartment 304. Sixty-two-year-old Isabel had lived in that apartment, with her twenty-one-year-old son, James, for six years. Apartment manager Virginia Tate trusted the mother and son to open and close the complex laundromat every day. They had known Paul for four years and considered him to be a friendly neighbor who kept mostly to himself. They had never seen him become violent or aggressive.

That was until the evening of December 14, 2000, when loud pounding, so hard their windows rattled, was heard at their door. James put the chain on the door and opened it. They recognized their neighbor at once.

"Paul, quit pounding," James said. "Go home."

Paul grunted and pushed an object into the door.

"Ma, he has a knife in his hand!"

Paul began to push to enter the apartment. The thin, 135–pound James yelled for his mother's help, fearing that Paul would break the chain off the door. Together, James and Isabel pushed the door shut and locked it. But Paul kept pounding, and a new sound suggested that he was also striking it with a knife. Photographs would later reveal scratch marks on the door, although it was unclear how old they were or if they were made that evening.

Isabel called 9-1-1

Two Lake Hefner rangers, one twenty-one years old and the other sixty-two, arrived at the complex. Officer Jeffrey Rooks, a twenty-six-year-old who had been on the Oklahoma City police force for a little more than a year, also arrived on the scene. Isabel and James were told to stay in their apartment.

The door to Paul's apartment was open, and a man could be seen sitting in a chair in the living room.

The officers called out, "Paul!" He motioned for them to come inside. One officer said Paul also invited them to "come on in," but in a low, "demonic" voice. Paul's first reaction to seeing Rooks's badge was to call the police officer a "jackass" several times. He muttered some other unintelligible words that no one could understand. At least two of the three first-responders spent time alone in the apartment with Paul. One news report would later say ten minutes, others a shorter amount of time. Whatever the length of the encounter, it would be the final minutes of Paul's life.

Chapter 26

The Cold Reality

"What did you just say?"

I was responding to the gravelly voice on the other end of the phone call: Virginia Tate, property manager of the Park Manor apartment complex, where my brother lived in Oklahoma City. Tate's voice was emotional, coupled with a sense of urgency. She repeated what she had just said.

"Joe, you have to come to the apartment now!"

"Why, what's wrong?" I said.

"The police have shot Paul!"

Her words did not process. I tried to grasp what she was trying to convey. As a journalist, I had learned to suppress my emotions during the worst of tragedies, but my hand was shaking as I held the phone waiting for Tate to tell me anything that would give me a glimmer of hope that my brother was still alive.

The remnants of the winter storm had more than doubled my usual twenty-minute commute home from work that day, and conditions were miserable. But I had traveled in a warm, dry vehicle, vastly different from the ten years Paul had slogged outside in the middle of the night to sand roads during snowstorms in his ODOT job. Arriving home, I had settled into my favorite chair to see what the TV weather forecaster was saying about another approaching storm.

Then came the call. Another damn phone call. "Are you sure?" I asked Tate, and then the question I dreaded asking, "Is he still alive?"

"I don't think so. He's been lying outside of his apartment for hours."

The news pierced me. The thought of my brother's body lying discarded outside for hours was almost more than I could take. I summoned the coping skills that as a journalist had seen me through the Oklahoma City bombing and the Moore tornado and so many other tragedies, and I yelled to Nan: *We need to leave right now! Paul has been shot by the police!*

* * * * *

The three members of law enforcement summoned to Paul's apartment that night ranged in size from five feet four inches tall and a 150 pounds to six feet tall and a 174 pounds. So even at the age of fifty-seven and more than 225 pounds, my brother Paul would have been an imposing figure, despite that fact that Officer Rooks had city-issued body armor and pistol, the latter a Glock model 22 .40-caliber, with loaded high-capacity magazine. The handgun fired Winchester 185–grain hollow-point bullets that can cause extensive damage when entering the body.

Inside Paul's small apartment, the living area would have been crowded, even stifling. In Paul's state of mind, four men in such tight quarters would have felt like being inside a pressure cooker, and the officer knew it. Rooks left to call a mental health officer from the Oklahoma County sheriff's office. He left the two lake rangers inside trying to calm Paul down. In a matter of seconds, what had been a situation under control went horribly wrong. For reasons unknown, according to reports, Paul got up—somehow evaded the two rangers—and made it into the kitchen where he grabbed a knife. He ordered the rangers to leave his apartment. One report said he backed them out. Another said they ran out.

Once out, the rangers closed the front door behind them to keep Paul contained in his apartment. No one would ever know what Paul was thinking in that moment. The only thing certain was that Paul did not want to be taken to jail, to the crisis center, or to any mental institution.

Police later said Paul came out his front door waving a fourteen-inch kitchen knife with a serrated blade, longer than nine inches. He first approached the lake rangers, who drew their semiautomatic weapons, and then Rooks, who already had his Glock drawn and ready to fire. The officers yelled multiple times to drop the knife. Paul did not say a word. Three shots were fired. Paul fell to the ground almost on the doorstep of his own home. "Gunshot wound to chest," the death certificate would read, "Homicide."

He died with thirteen cents in his pocket.

Nan and I arrived there just after 9:00 p.m. with Nan in a company car. The flashing lights of the police cars bounced off the apartment buildings, illuminating them in the winter's night. I searched for Paul's bedroom window for any sign of activity. I had hoped that Tate had been wrong about what she had seen and that Paul had only been wounded and taken to the hospital just blocks away. I had not retained what she had said about Paul's body still lying outside.

As I approached the apartment, I was stopped by a police officer. "I'm Joe Hight. My brother is Paul Hight."

The officer called out on his radio that a relative had arrived. A police detective approached me. Nan and I were shown to the back of a police car parked across the street. The detective confirmed that Paul was dead, asked me whether we were okay, and then in a kind tone began to ask questions: What was Paul's history? Any previous incidents? Had I noticed anything unusual? I remember wishing that he had been the law enforcement official to approach Paul initially. The outcome that night might have been different.

I told the detective everything I knew, including that Paul had been shot by a Guthrie officer back in 1996. I felt I had no reason to withhold anything. I was in shock, naively thinking that whatever I said was to help Paul, not be used against him. The police would eventually find out his history anyway. The detective told me they would continue to investigate and then take the body away for an autopsy. He thanked me and gave me a phone number to call if we had any other information to add or questions. He told us to go home so we could contact our family.

With the police lights flashing behind us, I drove away awash in grief. Tears trickled down my cheeks. Nan tried to console me, but it was as if I was all alone in the car, lost in thought. Thoughts about the police interview. Thoughts about Paul. Thoughts that made me fearful of the police for the first time in my life. Somewhere on that agonizing ride home, I realized that no matter what we said or did in his defense, Paul would be found guilty. I knew the investigation would prove that.

By the next morning, I was already planning for Paul's funeral. The trust Dad had left for Paul ensured that it would be a nice one. I had begun to think about our family's response to the tragedy. I was angry—a grieving brother but always a journalist, one whose news organization, the largest in the state, would be covering the story. I quickly contacted my supervisor and removed myself from the story, except for providing Paul's photograph to a fellow editor who called later.

In any situation, the police shooting of a former priest would create front page headlines and round-the-clock coverage, but Paul's case had the potential of creating a feeding frenzy, given that the police department was already under scrutiny for the rash of police-related shootings. I asked my sister Marilyn to serve as the family spokeswoman, knowing she would handle the inquiries with grace.

I began another family obituary, along with a family statement with my brothers' and sisters' approval. In my shock, I forgot that Paul was still fifty-seven; he hadn't celebrated his birthday yet. That would have been December 27.

The statement "Submitted by Joe Hight, brother of Paul Hight, on behalf of his five surviving brothers and sisters" was as follows:

> Our family is deeply saddened by the death of Paul
> Hight. Paul was 58 [sic], the oldest of seven children, a
> former Roman Catholic priest and a person who cared

for his family and friends. He was a kind and gentle man who was always giving away anything he owned to people who were less fortunate.

However, Paul suffered from a mental illness that afflicted him for nearly thirty years. How that affected Paul was difficult for anyone, even his family members, to understand. We did know that Paul had taken monthly shots at an Oklahoma City mental health-care clinic in an effort to silence the voices that haunted his life. In the last five years, there had been no serious incidents involving Paul and his illness. He wanted to live independently and did so during the final years of his life. He sought to help people who suffered similar maladies.

We don't pretend to know what happened Thursday night. And we deeply respect law enforcement and understand that they need to protect the community and themselves. We never wanted anyone harmed because of Paul, especially when his mental illness controlled him. And we appreciate the kindness of police after his death.

However, we are troubled that another person with mental illness has been killed. It troubles us that three police officers couldn't control the situation without shooting a person three times and killing him. It troubles us that mental health officials didn't notify family members if Paul was having problems in November and early December, a year after his own father had died of cancer.

Family members saw him weekly. Many times, more than once. Family members had lunch with him the Monday before his death. He was talkative and happy. He had no violent tendencies. In the last five years, Paul realized that he had a devastating mental illness and had sought ways to control it.

We hope and pray that everyone, especially our police, will consider the plight of the mentally ill and learn

ways to control these types of situations without result-
ing in death.

By Friday, *The Daily Oklahoman* had published a front-page story that stated, "Police shoot, kill knife-wielding suspect." Paul was not
named, but the article gave the first details of the shooting. Police said
the neighbors had been arguing and that the officers had told Paul to
drop his knife "several times." By Saturday, local news stations were reporting on the shooting too. "Man with Knife Killed by Police/Incident
Started with an Argument, Police Say" read a story from the Associated
Press. That article reported Paul had answered his door with a knife and
threatened the officers. It also stated:

> This is the eleventh time this year that Oklahoma
> City police had fired in self-defense, and the fourth time
> in the last three weeks they have shot and killed some-
> one. Rooks was placed on routine administrative leave
> as a matter of policy.

One news station carried an official photo of "Jeff Rooks" in police
dress uniform. With his close-cropped hair, he looked young for his
age, as if he had just graduated from high school. The news account
also included a survey: "Local police have been involved in several fatal
shootings lately. What do you think?" Viewers could check one of two
responses: "Police are too quick to shoot" and "Officers must act to
defend themselves." Being from Oklahoma, with its proud military and
conservative heritage, I knew what most people would answer. After
receiving our family's statement about the shooting, the news station
changed the story's headline to, "Police Shooting Victim Had Mental
Illness/Former Priest Was Shot by Police." The narrative was already in
motion about how a mentally deranged person had confronted, lunged,
and charged the officers.

The Daily Oklahoman assigned crime reporter Ken Raymond
to the story. His report was headlined "Police kill mental patient" and

included an infographic showing that city police had shot nine people on the south side of Oklahoma City and two on the north side in 2000. Paul's shooting was the farthest north.

Raymond's story included interviews with the family and the police as well as comments from the apartment manager, who had been among those at the scene. " 'We never had a problem with him,' Tate said. 'He was a real nice guy. Paul has been friends with everyone here, as far as talking or just having a cup of coffee. That's just the way he was. . . . Were they right in killing him? No. There were three of them there. Paul wasn't a hefty guy; he was kind of slim. I asked the police today why they didn't wrestle him to the ground or shoot him in the arm. They told me that when they feel they are threatened, the law is *We don't shoot to maim; we shoot to kill.*' "

In the aftermath, the police became defensive again. The officer who headed the police training center, Lieutenant Rhett Brotherton, said officers are taught to avoid aiming for limbs. Instead, he said, they aim for center mass, basically the chest or stomach, where chances for survival are slim. Brotherton went so far as to demonstrate how quickly someone with a knife can advance on a police officer. He took the role of the person who had the knife, which would have been Paul. Raymond described the officer as "charging 21 feet across the room in less than 2 seconds." More precisely, 21 feet in 1.5 seconds. He described that as the "minimum safety buffer against an edged or blunt weapon." Any closer, Raymond reported, and police will probably start to fire.

Brotherton called Oklahoma City's high number of police-involved shootings compared to other cities a "statistical anomaly." He said he was more concerned that "this many officers are being attacked with deadly force" and less with those who had been shot and killed by police, including Paul. Raymond, however, reported no cases of "dead cops" in the six shootings since October 12. Of those shot by police, only one had been carrying a gun. Three wielded knives. One carried a chunk of concrete. One was unarmed. Of those shot, four were killed and one paralyzed. Raymond then asked Brotherton: *Should police consider nonlethal force in certain situations?*

"That's absurd," Brotherton replied. "Use a baton or your hand-to-hand techniques against a guy with a knife and you've got a dead cop."

Brotherton didn't mention that Tasers and other nonlethal devices were already being used by law enforcement, and neither did the story, although Brotherton's own police chief knew about them at the time. In an interview with KOCO-TV, Police Chief M. T. Berry said police had been looking into nonlethal weapons, or as police called them "less-than-lethal weapons," over the past six months. They already had pepper spray and batons, but Berry mentioned the possibility of acquiring long-range nonlethal weapons that could disable a person but keep the person alive.

"You look at the recent shootings that we had," he said, "we have to go back and look at the situations to see if any of these (nonlethal) weapons might have been effective."

* * * * *

By Sunday, the same photo of the smiling Paul from news reports was used for his obituary in *The Oklahoman*, one of thirty-three paid obits toward the back of the paper's A section. The obituaries commemorated doctors, attorneys, insurance agents, oil company executives, housewives, ministers, a computer graphics designer, veterans, and an out-of-state newspaper editor and reporter who had worked in Oklahoma at one time. The youngest was thirty-one; the oldest, ninety-three. They were said to have died, expired, passed away peacefully, went to be with our Lord, her Lord, or the Lord she loved, or were called home to Heaven. Many had died of cancer, after a brief or lengthy illness, or simply of old age. Only one obit that day carried the words "died suddenly," but it didn't say the death was caused by gunshots from a police officer's weapon. And I wanted to make sure this obituary was different.

Paul Wilber Hight was known for his laughter. His gentle spirit. His giving ways. His love of God, family and friends. Those who knew him will remember those qualities when they celebrate his life on earth this week. Throughout his life, Paul remained devoted to God and the Catholic Church. His apartment was filled with Bibles and religious books that he studied and rosaries that he used to pray. He also continued to give to others, even though he didn't have much to give. And he loved to spend time with his family and friends; he usually greeted each one warmly and laughed loudly at their stories, even those that were not so funny.

The obituary said his funeral Mass would be held the following Tuesday at Saint Mary's in Guthrie. Marilyn was prepared again to serve as a family spokeswoman.

Two TV stations showed up for the funeral. One filmed inside and the other outside. Each person who came in received a card with Paul's favorite hero, Jesus Christ, on the front. The Lord's Prayer was on the back, with Paul's birthdate and date of death.

The front page of *The Oklahoman*, one of the only metropolitan newspapers that still carried a daily prayer on its front page, published a prayer that seemed to reflect the day on that Tuesday.

Dear Lord, many of us have endured great pain in our lives, be it emotional or physical, and at times there is no reprieve. Lift our pain, dear Lord, when it is too much for us, Amen.

Besides the TV reporters, more than a 140 people packed into Saint Mary's for the funeral Mass. Some of them had attended Paul's ordination more than thirty-two years earlier in the same church with the altar built by our father. They were my friends, friends of my brothers and sisters, friends of my parents, and Paul's friends, including Jerry Lindsley and Mary Wheeler. Five were nuns. Two were former priests, including Joe Thompson. Barnarda Sharkey, who would "miss his gentleness," was there. Members of Christ the King Catholic Church were there as well as people we didn't know or recognize, who might have seen the coverage on TV or read the stories about Paul's death and decided to attend.

Paul's friend Father Hanrahan officiated. Father Joe Ross, who had married Nan and me, delivered the sermon. But most surprising were the many priests who showed up for the Mass: Father Petuskey. Father Beckman. Father Stieferman. Father Morgan. Priests we did not know.

"Paul was loved by the priests," Stieferman said. "We all kind of felt like he hadn't been supported. That's why a lot of priests showed up. Father Hanrahan was the most upset." Maybe even more surprising was who led the priests: Oklahoma City Archbishop Emeritus Charles Salatka and Archbishop Eusebius Beltran. The procession of archbishops and priests reminded me of Paul's ordination when I was a child.

"All of the priests admired and respected Paul," Beltran would say years later. "I admired Paul. He had a tough time dealing with life. He suffered tragedy in death. I felt he was a kind, good man."

I had selected Father Ross to deliver the homily. With his gentle eyes and demeanor, he had a voice that could soothe the rage of some people who felt Paul had been killed unjustly because of his mental illness. Father Ross also had perfect recall of what had happened and what should be said that day. But even his words would become controversial.

Ross started with an analogy he had developed the year before. He described a neighborhood filled with trees. He told of how people in that neighborhood did everything they could to care for the trees. They watered them. They trimmed them. They used wire and cloth to tie the trees to stakes so they would grow straight. The same, he said, should be done for those who are wounded.

"We need to take care and reach out to someone who is wounded as you would in caring for trees," he said. "There's evidence of caring when you do something for a tree. The same with those who are wounded. There's humanity there."

Years later, he said he had images of Paul in his mind at this point: One of Paul as a priest. One of Paul with the dazed look of mental illness upon him. Then he made a statement that some of his fellow priests doubted. "It was odd, strange." Stieferman said afterward, and others would later say they were puzzled by it too.

He said the situation was traumatic for police too. That half of officers quit the police force after shooting someone. That they have regrets. That it was just as difficult for them. "We need to pray for the police who were involved in this," he said. "Pray for them as they wrestle with the trauma they have to deal with."

The church fell silent as he talked.

"I had memories of it—a feel for it," he would say to me after retiring more than fifteen years later, with Parkinson's disease consuming his body. "It was sad, but I knew there was tension. It was a loaded situation. It was hard for the family. It was hard for police. It was hard for you. I knew it was personal" for the police officer. "I wasn't saying it to excuse the police. It was just a difficult circumstance for them too."

After the Mass, Father Hanrahan led the final service for Paul. The sun had risen, and the temperature had climbed above freezing as we arrived for the graveside service at Summit View Cemetery. Paul would be buried next to his grandparents on the Hight side in the same family plot, along with Mom, Dad, and Linda, although I knew Paul would have said he was not in the cemetery, only his body.

Within two days, another man was shot and killed by Oklahoma City police after a bizarre chase involving a stolen car and a knife that had started in the town of Shawnee, thirty miles to the east—the twelfth police-involved shooting, the seventh since October 2000, and the fifth person killed. Oklahoma City police were less defensive this time. During the chase, one spokesman, Captain LaNell White, had told the media that police would try to control the situation if they could. "No one wants to take someone's life," he said.

Oklahoma City Police Chief M. T. Berry admitted to the media that he was concerned about public perception in the aftermath of so many police-related shootings. Two years before, Berry had been the first African-American named as police chief in Oklahoma City. He had been chosen from more than thirty other applicants, including five in his own department.

Chief Berry called FBI special agent in charge Richard Marquise and offered to let the federal agency investigate the shootings. Berry indicated that internal investigations into police-involved shootings had slowed because of the high number since October. The FBI were already investigating the death of thirty-eight-year-old Randle Carr, who was shot while threatening police with a chunk of concrete. However, Marquise seemed doubtful that anything would come from the investigation.

The FBI would collect police reports, interview witnesses, and gather what Marquise called "evidentiary reports" and then send the information to the Department of Justice in Washington, D.C. The justice department would decide whether a full investigation would be needed or if any of the evidence warranted prosecution.

"Typically, that occurs in less than 3 percent of the cases," the agent said. When pressed about this, Berry became defensive again. "I don't know why so many people are putting officers in a position where they have to use deadly force. . . . I share the concern of the public in that respect."

Berry's statement made sense at the time for a police chief, but what he did not address was that at least one of those people was killed while suffering a psychotic episode—not for any intentional criminal act. Because he had paranoid schizophrenia, Paul had one strike against him the day he began to show symptoms. Because he had been involved in a police-related incident in Guthrie, despite having been unarmed, he had another strike. The third strike was all but inevitable the moment he stepped outside his apartment door, supposedly with a kitchen knife. Police and the district attorney would investigate, but the case might as well have been closed as far as they were concerned.

But it wasn't closed for me.

Chapter 27

Justifiable Homicide

Sometimes when people think a saga is ending, they find that the story is just the beginning for others. That December shooting ended my oldest brother's life. I have no doubt, however, that Paul would have looked at it as the beginning of an everlasting life. For me, his death was also a beginning. It raised not a single question but many questions about the tragic circumstances surrounding his life and death.

In the case of a person killed by a police officer, the process is a difficult one. The family faces a justice system that almost always stands behind the officers involved; a public that wants to support the officers who protect them; and a societal belief that the person whom officers confronted was at fault. In investigative files, the case is tabbed as "Crime: Just Homicide" meaning justifiable homicide. The person shot by police is identified as a suspect. The police officer who fired the deadly shot or shots is the victim. That perception has been ingrained into our psyche by Hollywood and the media: the psychotic killer who's less than human, a danger to us all.

For family members, however, that person was human.

For me, that person was my brother.

For my daughters, that psychotic killer was their kind, happy, and generous uncle and godfather.

Most deaths end their public period with the obituary in the local newspaper and the coffin being lowered into the ground. That was never going to be the case with Paul's death. No matter what we did, we couldn't escape the escalating controversy.

And so we watched our oldest brother/uncle/brother-in-law die over and over on local TV and in the newspaper stories, always wondering: Would some good ever come from what we thought was his unnecessary death?

The Daily Oklahoman ran a lead editorial entitled, "Deadly Force/Threat Response Plan Should be Reviewed." The editorial defended police and repeated Police Chief M. T. Berry's assertion that the seven people shot by police in the city since October 1, 2000, had made a choice to come at police with a weapon.

> The fact that the seven shootings have occurred in a short period of time is not necessarily significant. It could be more a matter of coincidence, just as the number of state executions scheduled for January is coincidence rather than a calculated pattern.

But then the editorial added:

> What is troubling about these incidents is that they mostly involved the threat to the police from someone wielding a weapon other than a gun. In one case it was a chunk of concrete; in several other cases, knives were involved. Obviously, concrete and knives are no match for firepower. The police responded with superior force.
>
> We do not imply criticism of police with these comments. It is by no means clear that excessive force was used given the circumstances. Having said that, we believe it may be time for the police to scrutinize their

response to such deadly threats. Perhaps more directed and intensive training in this area is needed.

The top letter to the editor put it more bluntly: "City cops shooting to kill" was the headline to the letter written by an Oklahoma City resident identified as T. B. James. James asked what was wrong with the Oklahoma City Police Department. An excerpt read:

> It's turning into a "killing field" out there! The first response to a situation is gunfire?
>
> I understand that police sometimes must take extreme action with confronting extreme situations. But a woman with a knife, a man with a rock and a 58-year-old [sic] ex-priest with a knife. Think about it. Was shooting necessary?
>
> Use more discretion. Throw a net over them, use a Taser, negotiate or even wait them out. . . . Deadly force should only be used after all avenues have been exhausted.

Subsequent letters defending police were written, including one with the headline: "Police gunfights justified." Two others were written by an Oklahoma City police sergeant and an attorney who admitted that she and her law partner had defended police officers who had been sued for alleged civil rights violations. The headlines of those two letters, also the top ones on the page, read "Recent shootings justified" and "Police finest in the land." Both attacked James as ill informed and "biased in ignorance." They repeated what had been stated numerous times in the past—that it was troubling to them that so many officers had been attacked. Susan Knight wrote: Police officers are routinely placed in life-threatening situations in which their responses must be quick and sure, relying on their training and experience.

Knight, an attorney from Norman at the time, would later defend a police sergeant who pointed a gun at his grandson's father while off duty and then resigned right before pleading guilty to a firearms charge.

There's absolutely no indications that the officers in the recent shootings did any less. In each instance, officers' lives and the lives of citizens were threatened. We can all second-guess the actions of others in hindsight, I suppose, but James wasn't there. I have no reason to believe James has any police training or background whatsoever. If James happens to be attacked by a violent mental patient or drug addict, I wonder who he or she is going to call for help.

After Paul's death, we received numerous calls, emails, and letters of condolence. Masses were said for Paul throughout the metro area. I knew people didn't know how to respond in a situation such as the one we were living through. I was confused myself about what exactly to do, for my children, my siblings, Paul's friends.

I returned to work on December 27, 2000, Paul's birthday. There would be no celebrations this year. And the icy, cold weather had returned. I tried to stay in my office at *The Oklahoman* and kept to myself as much as possible. Many people took off the week between Christmas and New Year's anyway. I had time to catch up.

On my second day back, I received an email of condolence from Elana Newman, an assistant professor of psychology at the University of Tulsa in Tulsa, Oklahoma. She had worked with me at the Dart Center for Journalism and Trauma. A couple of hours later, she wrote again to offer any help for my "family in this time of shock, confusion, grief."

She seemed to know all the emotions that I was going through at the time. But she also wrote that she had called the home of the head of the Mental Health Association in Tulsa to tell him about what had happened to Paul. She wrote that he would be happy to consult with me.

"I thought of him since he has experience in working with mental health consumers and police, knows the ins and outs of Oklahoma policy about training police, mental health consumer needs and their families, knows advocates close to you that might be helpful," she said. "I also trust him deeply . . ."

That person was Michael Brose. I filed the email away thinking I would call Elana later in the week. I didn't want to talk to a mental health professional, particularly one from Tulsa, given Paul's history in that community.

A short time later, the phone buzzed in my office. During Paul's life, phone calls had usually brought bad news. And when you're in the news business, such calls are usually from people complaining about the bad news. I thought about letting the call go to voice mail. No one would have questioned me if I had. In hindsight, that might have been the best thing to do, in hindsight. Instead, I picked up the line.

The voice on the other end was Michael Brose, or Mike as most people call him, the executive director of the Tulsa Mental Health Association and a tireless defender for those suffering from mental illness. He mentioned that he had talked to Elana and had read the stories. *What happened?* he asked.

I told him what I knew about Paul and his life with mental illness. He told me how people with mental illness, especially paranoid schizophrenia, can become agitated and react to the command voices that police are taught to use in such encounters. "What happened was preventable," he said. "What they did was wrong." His words penetrated my shell. That and what was announced the same afternoon.

Oklahoma County District Attorney Robert Harold "Bob" Macy might have been among the last of the Oklahoma prosecutors with a Wild West sense of justice. An ardent defender of law enforcement and justice, Macy took pride in sending murderers to Oklahoma's death row during his career. He counted fifty-four such sentences in his twenty-one-year career. He looked the part of a prosecutor, a character straight out of those cheap dime novels about the American West. He lived on a ranch in Newalla, east of Oklahoma City. He liked to rope calves and steers when he wasn't prosecuting criminals. He decorated his office with drawings of cowboys. According to a story about his death November 19, 2011, in *The Oklahoman*, a poster from the movie *Tombstone* hung on his office wall, with the words "Justice is Coming" emblazoned across the top. Given Macy's reputation, I wasn't surprised that a decision on whether to prosecute anyone in connection with Paul's death was issued in only two weeks. At least the investigation lasted longer than the two days following the Guthrie shooting. Paul had gone in with three strikes against him anyway. In a letter to Chief Berry, Macy wrote:

> Our review of the facts of this case reveals that the use of deadly force by Officer Jeffery [sic] Rooks was justifiable under the Constitution and the laws of the United States and the State of Oklahoma. Use of deadly force by a police officer who is in the performance of his legal duties and when there is a reasonable belief that it is necessary to protect himself or others from serious bodily injury or death is legal under the laws of the State of Oklahoma. We decline prosecution against Officer Rooks for his justifiable use of deadly force.

The superlatives and phrasing were classic Macy and recalled the sounds of frontier justice. Macy wrote that Paul had been "waving the knife in a threatening manner from side to side" at the lake rangers and then had turned away and begun a rapid advance on Officer Rooks, "swinging the knife toward him in a life-threatening manner." Paul "ignored all verbal commands given by the officers." He came at them at a "rapid pace," again "with the knife swinging in a life-threatening manner." Macy mentioned twice the nine-and-a-half-inch serrated blade on the knife. He then concluded that the officer "feared for his life" and "was justified in using deadly force to stop the threat to his life."

That didn't anger me.

What did was the following paragraph:

> During the subsequent investigation, it was discovered that the suspect was Paul W. Hight. Mr. Hight had a long history of mental problems. In 1995, Guthrie Police were forced to shoot Mr. Hight in a similar incident. Through interviews with other witnesses, it was

discovered Mr. Hight had been exhibiting strange behavior indicative of being off his medication days before
the December 14 incident.

I then remembered my conversation with the detective in the back
of the police car. How I had told them about Paul's incident with police
in Guthrie. That we had taken Paul to get his shot that week. That my
brother had had mental issues in the past. I realized those "interviews
with other witnesses" included me.

Or as I thought at the time, possibly only me.

Michael Brose's words to me returned: Paul's death might have
been preventable and was wrong. I thought about what Brose had said
about command voices—our father had a drill sergeant's command
voice, one that often had caused Paul to become agitated and angry.
My only negative encounter with Paul had been when I tried to use
that same command voice. It was well known that police officers also
resort to a declarative command tone in such situations. That's how
they are trained. Most of the time, in most situations, the command
voice works. But as Brose said, the command voice does not work well
with a person who suffers from paranoid schizophrenia and is having a
psychotic episode.

Then I wondered: What had happened during those ten minutes
when the three officers first approached Paul in his apartment? I needed
more answers, beyond the quick resolution that Macy had made of the
case. I needed help beyond my journalistic abilities. I started to ask for
names of attorneys who had defended people in cases involving police. I
was given the name of Michael Taylor, a U.S. Army veteran and former
prosecutor based in Oklahoma City.

I called Taylor before New Year's. He didn't give me much hope that
what he might find would change anything, but I told him that didn't
matter. I wanted to know—I needed to know, my family needed to
know—what had happened. I persuaded my brothers and sisters to use
the remainder of the trust money Dad had left for Paul's care to hire an
attorney. I would pay any remaining amount.

By January 3, 2001, Nan and I'd had our first meeting with Taylor. Because of the media coverage, he was aware of Paul's death and the allegations. By the next Saturday, I was letting Dennis Berglan of Trace Detective Agency in Oklahoma City into Paul's apartment. Berglan and Earl "Butch" Simpson would spend the next month investigating the scene, interviewing witnesses, and obtaining any pertinent information they could find about the case and relaying that to Taylor. We would then receive the information via letter or in a file from the attorney. The detective agency filed its investigative report on February 13, 2001. The detectives had found several inconsistencies in earlier accounts by police and the district attorney's office. Based on their interviews, here's what they believed had occurred after the officers' arrival at Park Manor:

> The next-door neighbors thought the police had arrived at 7:15 p.m., five minutes after they had called them. By that time, the mother and son had pushed a couch up to their door in fear that Paul might get into their apartment. They told the police what Paul had done. "Stay in your apartment, away from the front door and window," one of the officers told Isabel and James, and so they had gone into their kitchen to wait. They were confused by Paul's actions because Paul had never shown any violent tendencies. While [Isabel and James] waited in the kitchen, they paged a "Mr. Cheatwood," identified as the Park Manor Apartment maintenance manager, saying they were having problems with Paul. He and his wife were at the nearby Penn Square Mall and immediately started back to the complex.
>
> Twenty-five-year-old Tamara was upstairs in her apartment watching TV. She suffered from a form of muscular dystrophy. George was her next-door neighbor. Mike was doing his laundry in the communal laundry room across from apartment manager Virginia Tate. He

returned to his second-floor apartment. He remembered looking at the clock. It said 6:50 p.m. He wanted to make sure because he wanted to retrieve his laundry.

A short time later, Isabel and James heard "Drop the knife" or "Drop your weapon" at least four times. Then they heard three shots. James opened the door to see Paul lying on the ground with two spent gun cartridges nearby. He also heard an officer say, "Close the door, and stay inside!" Others in the complex heard shots too. Mike was about to enter his bedroom when he heard what he thought was "six rapidly fired gunshots." He ran to get a baseball bat and left his apartment immediately to see what had happened. He could see part of the scene as he looked over the railing.

Tamara, moving slowly because of her muscular dystrophy, heard three quick gunshots and made her way to the balcony in front of her apartment that overlooked the swimming pool in front of Paul's apartment. George heard shots but stayed in his apartment for several minutes. Tamara went to the railing. She could hear Paul moaning and coughing. Then she saw one of the officers smoking a cigarette.

"Did you pick up the shell casings?" she heard one officer say.

Mike was now near the railing overlooking the pool. He saw one younger officer standing between two trees next to a rail fence on the west side of the apartment pool. He was looking at the sidewalk. Two other officers were at the southwest corner of the fence that surrounds the pool. They were looking toward Paul's apartment.

[Mike] screamed, "What are you doing!"

One of the officers by the pool said, "He had a steak knife." Mike moved closer to the railing. He saw Paul lying on his back at an angle to his apartment door.

His head pointed toward the pool, his left arm extended down parallel to his body, and his right arm extended out to the side pointing toward the pool. [Mike] did not see a knife. The officers were just standing there. "Are you going to help him?" he asked.

Moments before, Tamara had pounded on George's door. He came outside to find Paul on the ground. He could hear Paul moaning. He said Mike was yelling at the officers and upset because they were smoking. He remembered that he was upset because no one was helping Paul, and the officers were not doing anything. He heard radio traffic crackling near the pool, but none of the officers was talking on the radios. Mike then saw one of the officers at the end of the pool call the ambulance. About a minute or so later, he heard what sounded like a death rattle coming from Paul.

The Cheatwoods arrived at the apartment complex the same time as the ambulance, about two or three minutes later. They told an officer, most likely one of the lake rangers, that they lived in the complex. They were escorted in and saw Paul's body in front of his apartment door. His body was on the sidewalk with his feet in the dirt just beyond the sidewalk. As the Emergency Medical Services Authority personnel were being escorted to Paul's body, Mike heard one of the officers say, "He has a steak knife."

The EMSA staff members checked Paul and left the area. Mike still needed to get his laundry, so he went downstairs about five or ten minutes later. He was able to get close to Paul's body. He noticed Paul's shirt was open, and a large amount of blood was on his chest. Again, [Mike] didn't see a knife near Paul.

Paul's body remained on the cold sidewalk, according to some reports, for five to six hours. It was 27 degrees F.

outside. Isabel and James were taken to the police department at about 11:00 p.m. for separate interviews. They left at the same time Nan and I were in the back of the police car or just leaving the scene.

Later, Mr. Cheatwood looked at the wooden door of the next-door neighbors' apartment that Paul "had allegedly pounded with a knife." It had "very minor damage," he said, "that if the blows were struck with the knife, it would have been a small knife, and the blows would have (to) be struck with little force."

The maintenance manager also had to replace Apartment 306's window, which had been shattered by one of the police bullets that went into the apartment. It was fortunate that the person living in the apartment was not there at the time.

Berglan of Trace Investigations also tried to interview two other witnesses who had moved [away from the apartment complex] since the shooting. One didn't want to talk.

After seeing the report from the private investigators, Michael Taylor wanted more details. He wanted to see the actual homicide file.

Chapter 28

Priest Forever

Immediately after the shooting that ended in Paul's death, the police began the official investigation. They canvassed the neighborhood and interviewed at least twenty-four people, some multiple times. The department would eventually file a nearly 150–page report with interviews, detailed descriptions, and photographs of the scene, the complete file from the police-involved shooting in Guthrie, and the district attorney's own three-page letter justifying the shooting. The report also included interviews with officers and the ambulance crew and even minor reports about when various officers, in addition to the three original first responders, had arrived at the scene.

One officer wrote that she had responded at 6:49 p.m. to an officer-involved shooting at the Park Manor Apartments. Rooks and Sergeants Marang and Bach said they arrived at 6:43 p.m. and didn't leave until 8:55 p.m. Rooks said it took him five to seven minutes to get to the scene because of the icy streets and that he and the other officers arrived at the same time. A police lieutenant reported that the original call about the disturbance came in at 6:24 p.m., and the shooting was broadcast at 6:51 p.m., which was listed on the death certificate as the time of Paul's death. That all seems to correlate with what Mike, the tenant who was doing his laundry that night, said when he checked his clock at 6:50 p.m. as the shots were fired. The EMSA unit employees also stated that they arrived at the scene at 6:57 p.m., unzipped Paul's coat, placed electrodes on his chest, and then placed K-Y Jelly on his neck. However, they couldn't find a pulse.

That means Rooks and the other officers might have arrived more like 6:30 p.m. and had twenty minutes to talk to the next-door neighbors and Paul before the shooting occurred. The timing is important because of other reports that the officers spent ten minutes with Paul in his apartment. The times also seemed to contradict the final summary report that stated that officers had responded at 7:05 p.m. The next-door neighbors had told the private investigators that police arrived at 7:15 p.m., five minutes after they called. Other parts of the official report would contradict what witnesses would later tell private investigators.

> Rooks, interviewed at 9:00 p.m. December 14, 2000, said he responded to Paul as he had been taught in the police academy—to shoot within that twenty-one-foot area "in which a man with a knife could get to an officer and hurt or kill him. The man also accelerated his movement towards him while still swinging his knife back and forth. Rooks advised he felt he had no alternative but to use deadly force to save his life." Toward the end of the interview, the young officer said Paul was not breathing when he checked him and that he didn't want Paul to die. Yet witnesses say they heard Paul moaning in the immediate aftermath of the shooting while officers stood around smoking.

The two rangers told almost exact stories, but neither mentioned how long they were in the apartment with Paul before he went for his knife. They both said they had tried to calm Paul while Rooks was calling the county mental health officer, but neither provided what they had said to Paul or why he was allowed to get up from his chair and go to the kitchen where he was able to retrieve a knife. All three mentioned Mike with the baseball bat and said he continued to "verbally harass" or was "belligerent" toward the officers. One ranger said Paul was within fifteen feet of Rooks and then made a "sudden lunge toward him."

Beyond the officers, Paul's neighbors Isabel and James would be the primary witnesses to justify the shooting. The word *suspect* would be used continuously to describe Paul in nearly every witness account. However, one officer stated in his report that he "ran VI (victim) Hight FBI/OSBI through unit 800 with no record found."

James said he considered Paul a friend. Paul had given him a computer, which James couldn't get to work properly. Isabel said he had loaned her a quarter. "He was always friendly and always left his door open," James said.

Before the pounding on the door, the mother and son had ordered pizza and were watching *101 Dalmatians* on TV. James had arrived home at about 5:30 p.m. after a treacherous ride home from work on his bicycle. He had left the apartment for a short period to buy soft drinks from the apartment's laundry vending machine. They were fifteen to twenty minutes into the movie when they heard pounding at the door. James pounded on the table in the police department's interview room to demonstrate how Paul was pounding on the door. He said he opened the door and saw Paul with a black four-inch knife, although James also said it could have been some other sharp object. He later revealed that he had blurred vision in his right eye. James then called 9-1-1, and "the suspect left for fifteen to twenty minutes" before returning to pound on the door again.

Both James and Isabel said they were "really terrified," even petrified. Police asked Isabel if Paul had an interest in her. She said, "No." She described him as being five-feet-nine to five-feet-eleven and having a medium build. She said he smoked like a "fiend" and that his blinds were yellow from the smoke. Both Isabel and James said they had never had a problem with Paul before, but Isabel said she feared for her life that night.

"That wasn't Paul," she said James told her, "but it was like a man from a sanitarium."

Then Isabel made an admission that she said she "felt funny about making." She said, "In a way I'm kinda glad he's dead. Now I won't be afraid."

Police did find one witness identified as "Zary . . . from Iran" who had seen a man pounding on a door. "She advised that she never saw anything in his hand while he was hitting the door, but it sounded as if he had something in his hand. She said that the man was yelling and making a scene," police said in one report. "She told me that he was a very nice man and she never had any problems with him."

Police couldn't find anyone who had witnessed the actual shooting. Based on the weather conditions, that is not surprising. However, the absence of such a witness did leave continuing questions as to what had occurred in Paul's apartment and immediately thereafter. Mike, the witness who might have seen more than anyone else, was termed as "belligerent" and "harassing" to the point that he was deemed not credible. Police would write that Mike apologized for his behavior that night toward the officers but not before saying that he had heard the officers yelling for at least ten seconds before shots were fired and that the officer who shot Paul "was obviously in shock."

Mike wasn't the only one who questioned the police officers' behavior. Another James, who lived upstairs, said he was a college student who had been a "successful businessman" at one time. He also claimed he had lost his right eye from shrapnel in a war. Like Mike, he didn't know Paul either except to say he was a quiet person. James heard four or five shots and flashes at the window. He also went out on the balcony, and his was the voice that had asked. "Why did you shoot him? You didn't have to shoot him!" Mike had yelled at the officers too, becoming so outraged as time passed that James said, "He was getting a little out of hand."

Plenty of witnesses told police they had heard the shots, and some said that they knew Paul. They also said they heard the officers telling residents to "get back in your house." Another said she had heard a man yelling, "You guys shot someone last week!" or heard what Mike or James said they yelled at officers. A neighbor identified as Garreth said he ran out to see all the officers with their guns, saying, "Stay down, Paul. Don't get up, Paul." Some said they heard four or five pops "like someone banging metal," but others said six, and still others said "three shots fired in rapid succession." One said she heard two shots before 7:00 p.m. and ran outside to see two officers downstairs from her apartment who were joined a short time later by a third officer. Some who didn't know Paul cited his mental illness and called him lonely, strange, and an oddball. One had more than fifty samurai swords, medieval weapons, and what appeared to be a rifle in his apartment; he said he was afraid of police because a jailer had assaulted him at the county jail. He was afraid officers might shoot him because of his weapons. "I know why people rent Ryder trucks and why people buy fertilizer," the man said. "I helped police on a double murder at the fair too."

A fifty-four-year-old witness named Murray took three or four minutes to open his door slightly and then another five minutes before fully opening it and stepping outside to talk to an officer on the night of the shooting. The officer saw a "young white woman," about eighteen to twenty years old, on Murray's couch. The tall, slender man with graying hair claimed he was an artist and the young woman a model. He also told police he wanted to quickly leave the area, now swarming with police officers. He and the woman were later escorted to his blue Toyota pickup so he could do so. Officers took note of his license tag.

Many witnesses said they saw Paul walking back and forth to the Texaco station, one said at least fifty times. Others who knew him had other stories. Tamara said she saw Paul the day before and that "he was acting like the same old Paul. . . . Paul was a very good person." Karla said she saw Paul daily and that he was friendly and called her "Sunshine." She knew he had mental problems, but "it was very much out of his character . . . to cause a problem." Apartment manager Tate also said Paul had never caused a problem before and mentioned that he was a Section 8 tenant. She had seen him briefly a day or so before the shooting.

"Paul, are you feeling well?" Tate said she had asked.

"I feel fine," Paul replied.

Tate said that Paul had "told her in the past that his medicine did not make him feel good and that he felt better if he stopped taking the medicine," the report said. When asked whether she had ever contacted the family or NorthCare when she thought he was not taking his medication, she said she had not. That was probably because Paul had not caused any problems before.

The witnesses also included an Edmond commercial agent who worked in Oklahoma City. William called police on December 18 to tell them he had seen a man whom he identified as Paul from 12:45 to 1:00 p.m. December 14. The man was lying in the snow on the west side of the street near his apartment. "He slowed and that's when the man jumped up and ran in front of his car. He said he almost hit the man." Because of the icy streets, William slid his car to a stop. He said the man then ran to his car and laid down on his hood. "Run me over, please! Run me over!" the man told him. The man was not identified except to say he was wearing a jacket with no shirt, brown pants, and sandals similar to what Paul would be seen wearing later in the day. William said he didn't report the incident, "thinking the man was crazy or something like that." The officer had written on the report from William that it was an "officer involved shooting/justifiable homicide." That was ten days before Macy called it that.

Police took into evidence a "knife: 9" blade/4" handle-serrated bread knife" that they said Paul held in his right hand behind his lower back. A detective later said that he found Paul face up, with his right hand and forearm concealed under his back. Later, it was reported that Paul's body was turned over and the "14-inch knife had a 9½ inch serrated blade with a 4½ inch handle." Police also found a clothes hanger near Apartment 306 and "emory [sic] file/keys/paper" in Paul's front right pocket. They also confiscated from his apartment a bill from NorthCare, a two-year-old prescription bottle with twenty-one pills of Benztopine, used to treat Parkinson's and side effects of other drugs, a knife in a cutlery block, a knife in the kitchen sink, a kitchen knife in the bedroom, and an AT&T phone bill proving it was Paul's apartment. "It should be noted," the report said, "the entire apartment was very cluttered with clothes, miscellaneous papers, dishes, and trash. The apartment was very dirty in appearance."

No conclusions were reached on what exactly Paul was using to pound on the neighbor's door or if he had a knife then. As in the Guthrie case, it was assumed. Police also found the three shell casings "by the front door of apartment #304," the next-door neighbor's apartment. Paul's body was almost directly in front of his own door.

By the next day, the assistant medical examiner ruled Paul had died when one of the bullets "traveled through his heart and exited the back." He was also shot in the right shoulder, with part of the bullet exiting his body, and in the lower stomach area. The medical examiner also found "several bullet fragments from an old gunshot wound to the chest area."

The report also revealed that the gunshots never hit or grazed the arm of a man who had been reported as waving a knife back and forth or lunging at an officer. I would later receive the complete and extensive eleven-page autopsy in the mail from the medical examiner's office. It verified that the shot to the left side of Paul's chest caused his death but also stated that he could have survived the other two shots and that "toxicology was negative for ethyl alcohol and drugs."

Attorney Taylor kept pushing for more details. He had already written in a February 21, 2001, letter that "a number of inconsistencies remain. Crime scene reconstruction and witness interviews verify early reports that Paul Hight was shot within thirty-six inches of his front door. In addition, verbal commands the officers claim were given to Paul Hight several times to 'drop the knife' and 'to not come any closer' are inconsistent with numerous police department statements that the knife wielding suspect 'advancing,' 'continuing to advance' and 'advancing rapidly toward the officer.' I have also noted that while department statement's [sic] describe the officer's path of retreat as being blocked, physical evidence reflects otherwise. Finally, witness interviews indicate that the officers never attempted to render any aid to Paul after the shots were fired and simply directed paramedics to the body. . . ."

Taylor also insisted on seeing the file and crime-scene photos. During the first week of April, he was granted a chance to review them in the Oklahoma City municipal counselor's office. What he found was troubling and was recorded in an April 11 letter to my wife and me.

> The file was unorganized, and I observed several instances where handwritten notations had been whited out before the copies were made.
>
> No master index was provided with the file, and multiple page reports were out of order.
>
> The file contained hundreds of duplicated photographs but the numbering system used was not identified, was disjunctive and missing on many of the copies so no analytical analysis could be performed to cross check the information provided. Furthermore, the city would not provide any information on the internal review that was conducted following the "officer involved" use of deadly force.

In an annotation to the letter, Taylor wrote that Oklahoma City routinely conducts an internal review.

He then added:

> The most troubling aspect of the case revolves around the knife that Paul purportedly armed himself with before the shooting incident. None of the statements in the file address or explain how Paul managed to arm himself with this knife in the presence of two police officers. No step-by-step interview with any of the involved officers was contained in the file and their narrative statements do not detail these events. The knife issues became more troubling when I noted the lack of any crime scene photographs showing the knife. Don't get me wrong, there were a couple of photographs of

"the knife" but none of these were taken at the crime scene.

In all of the criminal and civil rights cases I have handled involving the use of a weapon against the officer, this is the first file I have reviewed that did not contain a single photograph showing the weapon and where it was located in the crime scene photographs.

Taylor then reached this conclusion:

I believe a young and inexperienced Oklahoma City police officer panicked when he shot Paul Hight as he came out of his apartment door. . . .

The location of Paul's body was on the apartment walkway directly in front of his apartment door. In the file I reviewed, this issue is glossed over by statements by all three officers at the scene that Paul first moved to the right down the walkway until shouts from the officer to his left caused him to turn an[d] advance toward that officer. What none of the statements explain is how Paul could have been advancing toward either police officer's position without ever leaving a walkway that did not lead to either police officer's location.

While I could spend a lot of time showing you that the Oklahoma City Police Department does not investigate officer-involved homicides the same way that they investigate all other homicides, the point is best simply made that they do not. . . . Challenging inconsistencies in statements and crime scene facts are the cornerstones for effective homicide investigations. When the goal is to vindicate, questions are simply not asked. Not only does the officer's original version go unchallenged, every effort is made to insure [sic] that the facts fully support that version of events.

Taylor recommended that we not pursue a civil rights case because "the City's potential liability would rest on a failure to train, screen, or properly supervise the officer, coupled with a showing that the officer acted unreasonably under the circumstances. Since all the officers were CLEET (Council on Law Enforcement Education and Training), that would be a "tough row to hoe." Furthermore, it is an open legal question as to whether or not the court would allow into evidence the shooting that occurred in Guthrie."

By that time, I had already decided not to pursue a civil rights case anyway. I did, however, ask Taylor to do one thing more: request a meeting with Police Chief Berry on how the department handles people such as Paul who suffer from mental illness. I told him that we wouldn't need to talk about Paul's specific case.

I couldn't change how Paul's life ended. Tragedy had stalked him for more than fifty years. Taylor's words couldn't erase the turmoil I felt about Paul's life and death. I had to find someone who could. And when I did, he was a Catholic priest who had been Paul's friend.

I took a seat on the couch next to his easy chair as Father Hanrahan as he rocked back and forth in his rectory next to Saint Mary's Catholic Church in Guthrie. He remembered his old friend Paul and the good times they had shared: the conversations, the camaraderie, those darn breadsticks that Paul liked so much. In those good memories, Hanrahan also included the times he had helped his friend as he searched for the words to console me. His face was lined with the wrinkles of old age, but his eyes shone with a youthful joy. He smiled at something in the distance that I couldn't see, and then the old priest turned and looked straight into my eyes. I knew what he was going to say before he said it: "Paul suffered much throughout his life, but he's in a much better place. I believe that. He believes that. As much as anyone who's lived on earth, Paul has earned his crown in heaven. For the first time in many years, he's finally at peace."

His words could have been my brother's.

All my life, I had heard Paul use similar ones to comfort me and others, including our own family after we lost Mom and Dad. Still, for those left behind, the idea of life beyond what we live on earth can be a concept that tests faith. We become like Thomas in the Bible, doubting until we can see to believe. When you're a journalist, that skepticism is ingrained in your DNA. We all want to be among the blessed who don't have to see to believe, but our human minds tend to get in the way.

Unlike my father, unlike Paul, in the aftermath of my brother's death, I did not turn to the Bible. I turned to some of Paul's writings from those notebooks of his. In one, Paul had seemed to find the answer to explain his own life. He wrote:

> *Jesus came to Earth not to destroy the law but to fulfill it. He did so by his crucifixion. Jesus, the sinless one, took the Penalty (Death) imposed by the Law because of sin upon Himself. Jesus suffered all the curses of the Law. So we might be free of them. . . . God sent His only begotten Son so that all who believe in Him might not perish but have eternal life. Salvation is not a matter of works, but a matter of Faith, belief in the Lord Jesus.*

He had jotted down Bible verses that supported this view. Then in his "principles for suffering," he seemed to write about his own life:

> *1. Suffering is necessary for all (Christ suffered). To be like Him, we must suffer.*
> *2. The end of suffering is eternal glory.*
> *3. Suffering is God ordained. God chastises those he loves.*
> *4. Those who suffer will achieve a crown of righteousness & glory.*

When under the influence of his disease, Paul could be one hell of a sinner, but when the medication or treatments or other steps quieted the voices, Paul was one hell of a saintly person. If he had been taken back into the Church as a priest, he might have been able to minister to people like him as well as others downtrodden by the capricious cruelty of this world. But for Paul, that wasn't meant to be.

In the end, one of the most important lessons to learn from my brother's story is that people with mental illness are people first. Paul had friends. He had a family who loved him. His life, as tormented as it might have been because of the mental illness, mattered. In how he lived, Paul showed that life is not about the lofty position you hold or don't hold but about how you live, how you influence the people in your life, the people who cross your path. Countless people crossed Paul's path, needing a quarter or shelter or a ride, and my brother was always there for them in their time of need.

As I drove home that day from Father Hanrahan's, I thought about the kindly priest's words, the many words I had read in the aftermath of Paul's death, and the many words that Paul himself had left behind—including some I found in a simple wooden box after his death. Handcrafted from walnut, the box was filled with words Paul had scrawled on tattered receipts and yellowed paperwork.

To my surprise, the box also contained a Christmas card from his old ODOT supervisor Garland Crabtree and a worn black leather pouch, or burse. The burse held an empty Holy Water bottle, an empty pyx (a container used to carry consecrated hosts for communion), and the words to administer the Last Rites and Sacraments. For my oldest brother, a priest who had been laicized, that burse and pyx represented his last enduring connection to the priesthood: the ability to administer the Last Rites to a dying person in an emergency. After polishing the tarnished canister, I found engraved on the pyx these words in Latin:

SACERDOS IN ETERNUM

The words translate to *Priest Forever*.

They echo the vow Paul took as a young man, and an abiding belief that must have made it so difficult for him to accept the Church's decision to discard him. I knew now that was also what some of his fellow priests believed too.

We say we value life, but I worried that I was alone in a world that failed to understand what Paul's life had meant to me, what it had meant to our family, what it had meant to so many others.

That night, I struggled to fall asleep. I lay awake thinking of what Father Hanrahan had said. I wanted to believe, but my mind kept getting in the way. Exhausted, I finally fell asleep with my doubts, and began to dream.

For centuries, humans have strived to interpret the meaning of our dreams—to determine whether they are signs from God, messages from loved ones from the other side, or a means to help us work through the problems we face. However, they might simply be a troubled mind trying to reconcile itself. In a way, my dream seemed to do all of that.

I was transported back to what appeared to be Saint Mary's, but this church had no statues of Jesus on the cross or Mary holding Baby Jesus in her arms. I was standing in the sanctuary as if I were an altar boy at a special mass. People I thought I recognized filled the pews. I felt a spirit of elation as if they were anticipating someone. A man in an ivory robe had his back turned to me, facing the congregation. His long hair flowed freely down his back. From the entrance to the church, a procession came. Priests. Bishops. Nuns. And then, people whom I was sure I knew. I saw my parents, young again, happy again, walking in front of a smiling woman and man who seemed the same age. I wanted to say something but couldn't. I couldn't hear anything either. I could only watch. And then I saw Paul, dressed in a simple white robe. The woman beside him had the cherubic face of Linda, the sister I never knew. Paul knelt in front of the man I couldn't see. He didn't prostrate himself. He didn't pledge allegiance. He had already done that in life. Instead, a simple gold crown, which I sensed symbolized eternal life and peace, was placed on my brother's head.

As soon as the ceremony had started, it ended. Paul stood and looked at me. The man in the ivory robe turned and did the same. I recognized him as the man whom I had seen years before walking near the highway with a cross, the man who had paused to tell me that everything would be all right. I had needed to believe that then, and I needed even more so to believe it now. The man smiled at me. So did Linda. So did my parents. But the widest smile of all was Paul's. The glow of his toothy grin filled the room.

I awoke with a smile on my face: My brother was finally at peace in Heaven. However, in the quiet of morning, I realized that I still had work to do—on his behalf and on behalf of all those who struggle with mental illness.

Until then, I could have no peace on earth.

Epilogue

The Fault of Our Systems

Author and writer Julia Dahl sat across from me in a hotel restaurant in downtown Oklahoma City in the summer of 2008. The hour was late, and the area, normally reserved for the hotel's breakfast crowd, was mostly empty except for an older couple chatting in a nearby booth. Dahl was in Oklahoma City to write a story about suicide by cop, or someone's intent to die in a confrontation with police.

To this day, I don't believe my brother Paul intended to die by a bullet from a police officer's gun, for many reasons, including his and the Catholic Church's beliefs regarding suicide. But also I remember his intensity about that Christmas list, and I'm sure he intended to see that list through. However, I felt it only fair that I meet with Dahl and answer her questions.

At one point during the interview, she asked me how I felt about the officers who had shot my brother.

"I've forgiven them," I said.

She seemed surprised. "That's not the usual response I get."

For me, that response had come after years of seeking to understand why police officers in two separate cities had felt compelled to shoot my brother. My original emotional response, which was to fear the very people whose motto is "to protect and serve," was gone. I had since met many police officers and law enforcement leaders through my work with the Oklahoma Partnership in Creating Change, an organization I helped form to bridge the gap between agencies and organizations that deal with those who struggle with mental illness. Many are caring and sensitive individuals. They want to find solutions to curtail tragedies involving people like my brother. I had come to believe, as Oklahoma County District Attorney David Prater told me during a one-on-one meeting, that an encounter with someone in a mental health crisis is a public safety issue for both the person with mental illness and the officer.

That path to common ground had started almost a year after my brother's death and the hiring of attorney Michael Taylor. From the beginning, my goal was not to sue someone but to find the truth about what had happened that night. I remember on hearing this that Taylor cut his fee in half and agreed to help us as our attorney.

As Taylor was completing his investigation, I asked for a meeting with Oklahoma City Police Chief M. T. Berry. In a letter dated June 12, 2001, Taylor delivered that request to a city attorney, Richard Smith:

> When you . . . arranged for me to review the homicide investigation file on the officer involved shooting of Paul Hight I told you my client had indicated an interest in meeting with the Chief of Police. A couple of days ago, my client contacted me and asked if such a meeting could be arranged.
>
> The purpose of this meeting is not to further investigate, review or criticize the involved officers' training or actions in connection with this incident. Nor are we questioning the department's investigation, findings or conclusions. As I am sure you can understand, my client is keenly interested in the way that law enforcement deals with the mentally ill when those inevitable

contacts arise. On May 21, 2001 the Oklahoma Legislature allocated a $12 million funding increase to be
earmarked for setting up a "Mobile Crisis Intervention
Team" in Oklahoma County. The idea is to provide law
enforcement with an effective alternative in situations
where they come in contact with a mentally ill individual who potentially poses a danger to himself or other
persons.

As a person who is typically cast in the role of criti-
cizing an individual police officer or department actions,
I find my part in this process to be somewhat refreshing.
I hope that you will discuss this with the chief and hope-
fully, help me set up this meeting. If handled properly,
such a meeting could provide the Oklahoma City Police
Department with a public relations bonanza and those
opportunities do not come along too often . . .

Taylor was referring to legislative action that some people were saying had been prompted by my brother's death. In newspaper stories,
Steven Buck, then executive director of the Oklahoma chapter of the
National Alliance on Mental Illness, had said a crisis team might have
been able to intervene in an encounter such as my brother's. Mental
Health Department spokesman David Stratten was quoted in a May
11, 2001, story in *The Daily Oklahoman* as saying of the shooting of
Paul, "That's the very kind of incident where a mobile team would be
called. I think the most important thing for family members who have
a loved one in this situation . . . they can call a mobile crisis team as an
alternative to law enforcement."

Later that year, the police chief granted my request for a meeting,
although it wasn't the "public relations bonanza" our attorney had pre-
dicted. On a morning in early November, I joined a delegation that
included Taylor, Buck, my sister Marilyn, and Anna McBride, a local
longtime advocate for people with mental illness whose son had had
altercations with police downtown at police headquarters. Chief Berry,

Captain Jim Fitzpatrick, then head of the Oklahoma City Police Crisis
Intervention Team, and a city attorney represented the police department. The meeting would be one of Taylor's last because he died three
weeks later at the age of forty-eight after a brief illness.

Nearly two decades later, Buck still recalled the meeting. "I remember an environment that was certainly tense," said Buck, who later became deputy commissioner for the Oklahoma Department of Mental
Health and Substance Abuse Services and then executive director of the
Oklahoma Office of Juvenile Affairs and eventually a friend of mine.
"The principals who had leadership positions displayed a demeanor of
not understanding what had happened nor an appreciation for what
should have happened."

Of the police contingent, Chief Berry was the calmest. He explained
what police faced when they confronted those with mental illness. He
pointed to how the department was learning about an increasing number of rural officials who were giving one-way tickets to residents with
mental illness so they would leave town and go to the metro areas such
as Oklahoma City for their social service needs. As he talked, I remembered the deal that the Logan County prosecutor had offered after the
first shooting involving my brother in Guthrie: move your brother out
of Logan County and do not file any legal action, and this office will not
seek any legal action against Paul. Later, Fitzpatrick discussed the CIT
program, which aims to end situations such as my brother's peacefully
and to train officers on how to maintain a nonthreatening posture in
such encounters. He maintained that the police department did not
take the action because of my brother's death, even though the program
was in the planning stages at that time.

The conversation was cordial and never accusatory, but it made me
realize the struggles police face with the ever-increasing number of people with mental illness who live independently in cities and towns, both
big and small, on the streets. How often officers must confront situations
that they are not prepared to handle—it didn't seem fair to law enforcement or people with mental illness. The only feeling I expressed during
the meeting was my belief that most officers were not trained properly

to handle situations or encounters with people with mental illness. After the hour-long meeting, Chief Berry stopped my sister and me in the hallway. "I'm sorry for the loss of your brother," he said. I felt his condolence was sincere. As much as I wanted answers, he wanted them too.

A few years later, Fitzpatrick became the president of TOPICC and an officer I deeply respect for his passion about what is needed to resolve this national crisis. The Oklahoma City Police Department supported the organization, especially under the leadership of Bill Citty when he was chief. TOPICC continued for several years but eventually began to falter. In 2012, I left for a new job as editor of *The Gazette* in Colorado Springs. I am back in Oklahoma now, and have spoken with the Mental Health Association Oklahoma about reviving TOPICC under a different name. It is still needed.

The day I spoke with Dahl, I still remembered the meeting seven years earlier with Oklahoma City Police Chief Berry. I assured her that although I no longer blamed the officers for the shooting, I did blame the system that eventually caused Paul's death, a system that had failed to properly train officers for when they encountered some of our most vulnerable citizens. The fact that in the twenty-first century, police were still required to have only one hour of mental health training annually—and could fulfill that obligation by watching a video on stress—was laughable given what we now know about mental illness and the massive deinstitutionalization of the past decades. The same indifference to people with mental illness also extends to the prison system.

No, I didn't blame the officers who shot Paul. I blamed a system that barely made the effort to pretend that it was trying to do better—that refused to even ask the questions that might lead to better results. "I realized these people weren't talking to each other," I told Dahl, adding that I did sincerely believe Paul would still be alive if a CIT team had been called immediately on that freezing December 2000 night.

Several weeks after the 2008 interview, I sat in a Chinese fast-food restaurant in Oklahoma City sipping egg drop soup while I read a report issued in October 1980 by Dr. Frank James, director of Management and Program Analysis for the Oklahoma Department of Mental

Health (now the Oklahoma Department of Mental Health and Substance Abuse Services), and Deputy Director Dick Gregory on the need for "Improving Psychiatric Care for Prisoners."

In their summary, James and Gregory expressed the following:

> While psychiatry has been ambivalent about treating mentally ill offenders, recent mandates for better mental health care for prisoners will require the profession's intervention. The authors, whose study of mental health care needs of inmates in Oklahoma, believed that because the prison is a community, a community-mental-health-like system offering a continuum of services is indicated. Some of the services they propose for prisons include outpatient and partial hospital services, an acute inpatient unit, a residential tertiary care unit, and an intermediate living unit. They also believe that mental health professionals should help improve the environment of prisons, and can do so by sharing lessons learned in their own institutional settings about the effects of a therapeutic community and a legitimate patient government.

The report stressed the growing demand for improved health care:

> Professionals and some courts who are familiar with the health needs of prisoners recognize that the greatest need is for psychiatric treatment.

The report cited the lack of psychiatrists in the state prison system.

> [A] factor most likely contributing to the lack of psychiatric involvement is the attitude of many prison administrators and prison caretakers; they often view psychiatry as a soft touch in a hard setting. Even the

blatantly psychotic inmate is first seen as *bad* and perhaps requiring more security precautions, and only secondarily seen as *sick* and requiring treatment and understanding.

As I read the report, I thought about how I had heard countless times that legislators were reluctant to provide funds for diversion and treatment because it made them appear soft on crime. James and Gregory had found the same in their study. That study is now among the many reports and recommendations that have been provided to public officials in Oklahoma and across the nation that have been shelved, tossed aside, or ignored. That attitude persists, and so the crisis still exists.

Living with Paul's story again as I wrote this book renewed my desire to push for improvements in how we care for and protect people with mental illness. But as I told Father Joe Ross after interviewing him, that couldn't happen until I went through the final stages of forgiveness. I had already forgiven the police, but I had others to forgive too. I had to forgive the mental health system for its many issues during Paul's life. I had to forgive the Catholic Church for how it rejected Paul in his time of need. I had to forgive myself for not being there in the moment Paul needed me most and for fearing people such as Paul who suffer from such a cruel illness. And I had to forgive Paul again too for leaving us just when he had become such a rock for my family. Such forgiveness was needed if I was to write with clarity about the demons that had stalked my brother, the illness that had consumed him, and the system that continued to ignore the plight of people who suffer from mental illness, thus helping to perpetuate the stigma surrounding it.

Throughout Paul's death and all that followed afterward, I had stayed calm and done what needed to be done next, even as the years added up. However, on June 11, 2015, after a conversation with a priest who was being forced to retire because of Parkinson's disease, I cried openly in my home office with my computer in front of me. I had tried to remain objective and unemotional through the trauma of my own life, but in that moment, all my defenses gave way: I grieved for the childhood I had spent in the shadow of Paul's illness. I grieved the loss of my oldest sister, whom I never knew. I grieved for the unnecessary loss of my oldest brother, the priest who didn't deserve to be discarded or to die the way he had died, alone in the cold with no one responding to his calls for help.

I had to grieve before I could begin again—before I could write the story I needed to tell. Several times after that, typing the words out on my computer or recalling a particular moment, the tears came. Facing my own words was emotionally draining; still I wrote. I wrote to fulfill what I believed was the difficult task that Paul was asking me to do in my dream—this book.

I told myself that I couldn't write another book until this one was finished. And I used the "theory of one" to justify it: If one priest is taken better care of in the future. If one person suffering from mental illness receives better care. If one person doesn't have to sit unjustly in a jail. If just one person is served, then this book, conceived many years after Paul's death, would have been worth the human cost to write it.

However, as I write this, the *ifs* have become all too numerous. The stigmas that existed during the 1950s, 1960s, and 1970s—almost forty years later—still exist, only now with increasingly militarized police forces. And the *ifs* that can make it difficult for a family to help even one of its own continue to multiply. One of those *ifs* is how records are shared with family members after the death of a loved one who suffered from mental illness. Privacy and the right to it are important. However, providers of mental health services to often seem to hide behind state and federal laws to deny records to family members even after the loved one's death.

The providers mainly use the Health Insurance Portability and Accountability Act, or HIPAA, along with a provision concerning the confidentiality of alcohol and drug abuse records called 42 CFR. Despite more than eight years of requests, NorthCare continues to refuse to provide records about Paul's treatment (based on a privacy law that did not exist when Paul was killed), despite three separate attorneys from ODMASAS, which contracts with NorthCare, saying they should be released. ODMASAS Communications Director Jeffrey Dismukes reasons that agencies like NorthCare are "fearful of repercussion," afraid that "they'll lose their jobs."

The only NorthCare record of Paul's that I've been able to obtain concerns an administrative breakdown stemming from one of Paul's procedures. And that came because of Dismukes. Paul came to North-Care for a "level of care change" and "information update" on July 11, 1997. Other than that, Paul had to update his information once in 1998 and twice in 2000. The last entry was "discharge—death" on December 14, 2000, the day he was shot and killed at his apartment. Medicare records indicate that Paul didn't visit NorthCare in November 2000, and no follow-ups apparently were made by NorthCare to ensure that he had received his monthly shot.

Oklahoma mental health providers, such as NorthCare, which contract with the state are supposed to do follow-ups, Dismukes said. "They get incentives. It's how they get paid." He said it had been a priority with his agency's current administration. However, questions remain about whether it was a priority with past administrations when Paul was alive or whether today, mental health agencies are building narratives about their patients to bill state agencies. One high-ranking state official who asked not to be identified questioned the outreach to patients such as Paul who are in the community and sometimes fail to report for their monthly appointments. In other words, could or should mental health providers report that patients are being seen when they are not? "Are they servicing the chronically ill to the level they need to?" the official asked.

For family members, trying to determine the level of care an ill family member in the past or present has received or is receiving remains difficult. Dismukes suggests going the route of guardianship or staying engaged in the treatment process. Our family, however, was engaged, and we still didn't know what was going on with Paul until it was too late. To make matters worse, many records that could help family members find answers are being destroyed. Some states require retention for ten or more years. For others, the window is much shorter. Again, states sometimes cite HIPAA, the act that was supposed to protect individuals, as an excuse for what they do or don't do as well as what they will or won't share with family. Dismukes thought many old records at Griffin Memorial Hospital in Norman and Eastern State in Vinita had been destroyed. "A lot of them are gone," he said, adding this glimmer of hope. "They may be sitting (in storage) somewhere."

Those records also might be important in determining possible abuses or deaths that have occurred in mental health institutions in Oklahoma and elsewhere. As stated in this book, two people I interviewed who stayed at Griffin witnessed abuse and unattended deaths. Fortunately, a safeguard has been put in place to prevent that. Dismukes said that his agency added an investigator in 2009 to investigate complaints of abuse and death brought to the attention of the department's board. That wasn't the case when Paul was alive or for thousands of other people who went through the system.

Records can help family members determine whether a preexisting condition triggered the onset of mental illness or possibly intensified it. In Paul's case, I found out through records and then in subsequent research and interviews that he had had a severe case of the mumps while he was in the seminary. Could mumps have been the reason that a person who had never showed signs of mental illness started to develop symptoms when he was twenty-eight years old? Our family would have never realized that might have been a possible trigger without those records. My father, mother, and Paul died without knowing it. If the Catholic Church had realized that Paul developed mumps while under its care at seminary, would the Church hierarchy have been so quick to laicize him after he started to develop symptoms?

I was able to obtain Paul's records only because I made the initial requests before 2010. A second check to determine whether any more were available turned up only an Excel spreadsheet noting when Paul went to a state or state-contracted agency.

As for the Catholic Church, a two-thousand-year-old institution known for its meticulous records, it uses canon law to keep such records secret. It took eight years before I received an outline and explanation about the contents of Paul's records, and that might have been only because of a new bishop and vicar general in the Oklahoma Church. I found it refreshing in 2017 that Tulsa Bishop David Konderla and Vicar General Father Elkin Gonzalez at least considered my requests and provided information I had not been able to get before. Then two years later, the diocese released twelve of forty-one documents that it considered "of public nature" from Paul's file. However, I could not make copies; I had to handwrite and type those files as a diocesan official watched me. Two of the "private" documents involved requests I had made to then Bishop Edward J. Slattery.

I am thankful that Father Gonzalez was responsive to my email requests and even sat down with me for a brief interview. He expressed a concern about what he considered the need to protect Paul and other priests from negativity, even after their deaths. I could respect that, but as a journalist who believes in transparency—and as a family member who wanted the facts surrounding my brother's laicization as they pertained to his untimely death—the need to know seemed more important, especially if that could save one person, even one priest, from what had happened to Paul.

There are small signs of a possibly more open Oklahoma Church. However, overall, the Catholic Church, facing continuing public relations crises, seems stuck in a system of denying or ignoring that its priests have problems. I contacted five of the largest U.S. archdioceses—New York, Chicago, Philadelphia, Boston, and Los Angeles—as well as the U.S. Conference of Catholic Bishops about how they deal with priests who suffer from mental illness. Only one returned my phone call, and most of the others didn't even bother to reply. If they did, the response was in the form of an email referring me to a mental health institution.

Although Church guidelines on priests who suffer from mental illness might exist, it's hard to determine what they are or how a family seeking answers in the aftermath of a family member's death would find them. Father William Grogan, the likable vicar for health care in the Chicago archdiocese, did tell me in a phone interview that the screening process for new seminarians has become much more structured, with candidates undergoing a psychological profile and screening before being accepted. Seminarians now are less likely to enter the seminary while still young boys, as Paul did when he was fourteen, instead, Grogan said most are in their mid-twenties. After I told him about Paul, he said he would pray for my brother, my family, and others dealing with similar situations. As for the Boston archdiocese, it supports a "Priests' Recovery Program for the education, intervention, rehabilitation, and pastoral care of [priests] living with alcohol and substance abuse." A staff assistant at the U.S. Conference of Catholic Bishops referred me in an email to three other places that also help priests in Maryland, Michigan, and Pennsylvania.

My research and interaction with the Catholic Church has led me to believe that canon law, the code of ecclesiastical laws governing the Catholic Church, is the root cause. Presently, canon law allows priests to be judged "unqualified" because of mental illness. If one in four members of the general population has some form of mental illness, then the Church might well have a similar number of "unqualified" priests who suffer from mental illness in one form or another. And canon law does not distinguish between those priests who have severe mental illness that makes them a danger to themselves or others and those who suffer from mild depression or some other diagnosis that can be controlled by medication. Canon law does not appear to hold the Church responsible for caring for those priests such as Paul who are diagnosed with mental illness during their priesthood either.

As noted in the beginning of this book, the Church is filled with saints who acted oddly during their lifetimes and were killed by authorities because of their behavior. However, the modern Catholic Church is bound by canon law that would have rejected some its greatest saints, and that flouts the 1996 writings of Pope Saint John Paul II, which said those suffering from mental illness "always bear God's image" and that "our actions must show that mental illness does not create insurmountable distances." I agree with what Archbishop Emeritus Beltran told me about the Church's approach to priests who suffer from mental illness: "There's a lot more concern today than forty years ago. It's not unusual for priests to get extended periods of rehabilitation." Father Gonzalez also referenced a priest he had dealt with who suffers from mental illness and been "treated in a different way" than might have happened in the past. He added that the type of laicization that Paul faced in the 1970s probably would not occur today. "It would be only requested if a person committed an action that was detrimental to others, such as child abuse," he said.

That is not to say that the Catholic Church does not have ministries for those with mental illness. Grogan's own Chicago Archdiocese has an Archdiocesan Commission on Mental Illness and Mental Illness Ministries. The commission provides "workshops and seminars for clergy, chaplains, seminarians, parish ministerial leaders, and anyone who will listen!" That outreach program is part of the National Catholic Partnership on Disability, which includes a section related to mental illness. But if John Paul II's words are to have lasting impact, the Church must also look inward and address how it treats its own people, its priests, who suffer from mental illness.

A statement from the Catholic bishops of New York would seem to reflect what Paul felt during his time on earth:

> In our society, those with mental illness are often stigmatized, ostracized, and alone. The suffering endured by mentally ill persons is a most difficult cross to bear, as is the sense of powerlessness felt by their families and loved ones.

New York is an archdiocese that didn't respond to my inquiry.

As for law enforcement, methods have improved on how they interact with people who are having psychotic episodes. Unfortunately, what that response is still depends too often on what officers respond and the training they have received. If anything is to be learned from the number of black men shot and killed in recent years by police, the takeaway had to be that police feared them. They were different. They have been demonized, as have people with mental illness. And although he was not black, Paul was a big man and someone to be feared when he was off his medication. He was also different.

Michael Brose points to only one city he believes has made significant progress in this area: San Antonio. The city was profiled in a 2016 *Boston Globe* story on how it has made mental health care a priority, with a "real system built with creativity, humanity, and sustained commitment." The mental health authority of Bexar County, the seventeenth largest county in the country of which San Antonio is the county seat, was on the brink of closure and had a $6 million deficit at about the same time Paul was shot and killed. Then a coalition of community leaders, law enforcement, government, mental health authorities, and others came together to divert more than one hundred thousand people from jail and emergency rooms, saving nearly $100 million.

Globe reporter Scott Helman wrote in that December 10, 2016, story:

> They have acted aggressively and spent heavily, confident their investments would pay off. They've done what many Bay State advocates dream of, and one thing those advocates resist: taking decisions on treatment and medication out of the hands of the most severely ill.
>
> All San Antonio police officers are required to take the forty-hour Crisis Intervention Training. The CIT program teaches police officers about mental health conditions, medications, and resources and trains them in oral deescalation skills. Traditional training teaches police to control situations by demanding compliance, and the unpredictable condition can be misinterpreted as a threat and quickly escalate to violence. CIT training is meant to prevent that.

An analysis by *The Washington Post* found that 124 of the 462 people shot to death by police in the first six months of 2015 were having mental health or emotional crises. That represents about 27 percent of those shot and killed, which correlates with the one in four of the general population who have some form of mental illness.

It should be noted that in both situations involving Paul, officers were modeling training that they had received—training that did not include or follow CIT. So when police departments say they train their police officers in how to deal with people who have mental illness, that only works if it is the right kind of training. The lack of proper training becomes a public safety issue for the officers and the people they interact with. Brose said he has been confronted many times by people struggling with a mental health crisis, and not once has any of the situations turned violent.

"Training teaches you that we're going to back up. We're going to buy time. Most people will calm down. That command voice training that [police are] given just doesn't work in these situations. If you're delusional, psychotic, paranoid, that doesn't work, and someone gets shot and killed. . . . usually the person who's ill," he said.

Law enforcement's "approach is to send our officers in harm's way without training and where the use of deadly force may be used in dealing with very complex situations. It's not fair to officers to respond to someone at a critical moment when a person is not thinking clearly, from anxiety or paranoia, and not to provide them with adequate training," Brose said. "Data shows a reduction in deadly force with training. It's been covered. They can fool themselves. They can fool the public. But they don't fool me anymore."

Without proper and detailed reporting of what happened in and outside Paul's Oklahoma City apartment the day he died, it is unclear how the two rangers tried to calm him down or if they managed to deescalate the situation at all. If they did use calming tactics, why did a person suffering from a mental health crisis feel compelled, as they say, to go to the kitchen and get a bread knife?

Although Oklahoma City deserves credit for increasing and improving its community policing programs when Citty was chief, the department still has issues with police-involved shootings. In 2013, six people were shot and killed by Oklahoma City police officers. An analysis by

The Oklahoman found that twenty-eight people had been killed and fifty others wounded in officer-involved shootings from 2004–2013; no police officer was killed in any of the incidents during that time. "Confrontations between officers and the public that end in gunfire are the most important cases a department can confront, law enforcement experts say," reporter Juliana Keeping wrote in the 2014 story "Deadly Force: A decade of Oklahoma City Police Department shootings" in *The Oklahoman*. "Such incidents can influence community perceptions and, if mishandled, undermine the credibility and public confidence in the police."

Police-involved shootings are so detrimental to public perceptions that one public official quickly said *no* when asked whether he would recommend Oklahoma City to someone living with mental illness. His answer was based on the possibility of the person being shot by police.

Nearly 51 million people are estimated to suffer from schizophrenia worldwide—2.2 million in the United States. I believe those who struggle with paranoid schizophrenia, like Paul, suffer more discrimination. The reason: The disease causes them to act belligerently, even violently, when pressed, surrounded, or commanded.

At one organization that helps people with mental illness, I was told that everyone is welcome except those who have violent tendencies. Since Paul's death, similar statements have been made to me countless times, even by people who I feel are the most sensitive about mental illness. The "built-in message and stereotype," as Brose calls it, also has been continually amplified by the media and Hollywood. Dismukes agrees.

"The huge issue is that we think that the crazies are going to kill people," he said. "People are still judgmental."

A gentle giant who suffers from severe depression with acute anxiety disorder himself, Dismukes now holds one of the top positions in the Oklahoma Department of Mental Health and Substance Abuse Services. He openly talks about a time when he tried to talk his way out of the doctor's office so he could kill himself. His doctor recognized the signs and stopped him. Instead of treating Dismukes as part of the system, the doctor "treated me as an individual." Could the Church not do the same?

Dismukes now sees his condition as an asset to his department, a stance his bosses have supported. Dismukes also notes the growing recognition of how substance abuse and mental illness are linked, both being diseases of the brain. Science understands that, but mental health and law enforcement systems seemingly still do not—or at least their policies do not reflect such an understanding.

"We need to talk about the fact that we're dealing with medical issues. We understand more. There are more interventions now. There's a focus on wellness. We're talking about getting well. We're talking about hope," Dismukes said. "Before," when Paul was still alive, "there was just a lack of hope. . . . just management of the disease. You were never to have hope beyond management."

Yet what is life without hope? Or gratitude, for that matter. Numerous studies, according to the *Harvard Mental Health Letter*, have shown that both are not only necessary for well-being but improve one's chance for being happy. Despite all he endured, Paul remained a grateful person until the end. In his own writing in 2000, the year he died, he wrote, "I was blessed spiritually, then physically, then financially, understanding He had been blessing me all my life . . ."

For those of us who have never suffered a paranoid schizophrenia episode, trying to understand what happens and how you feel when off medication is all but impossible. The only thing I can compare it to is a rage that fills every cell in your body, a little like how you might feel if a great injustice was committed against you. Most of us can control ourselves in such moments, but we don't have voices spurring us on or hallucinations adding a false narrative. With paranoid schizophrenia, the voices taunt you. The sight of a badge or uniform enrages you. The rage bursts out in unimaginable and unpredictable ways that frighten even the person who is out of control.

Years after Paul's shooting death, my older daughter, Elena, and I were heading home after a trip to watch the Saint Louis Cardinals play. She asked me a question, "How can you still be Catholic, knowing what happened to your brother and the history of the Catholic Church?" After a car accident stalled us outside Joplin, Missouri, on Interstate 44, my answer evolved into a long conversation about police, the Catholic Church, mental illness, and the mental health system. I told her the Church was built by fallible people who had made and would continue to make mistakes. It had always been so, and, yes, that had led to some dark periods in the Catholic Church over the course of its almost 2,000 years, but the living Church was a personification not of man but of a loving God. My faith was instilled in me by my mother and father, and, most important, by Paul himself.

"If my brother went through the hell he did and still had faith, then so should I," I told her.

That faith gives me hope that caring people within those systems will change them. That one day we will overcome the stigma that impacts the people amongst us who live with mental illness, millions of people—people as close as your aunt, uncle, niece, nephew, sister, mother, father, or maybe even yourself.

Or maybe your oldest brother, a Catholic priest who had to suffer an unnecessary death because change didn't come soon enough.

A Final Word

For Now

"Blessings." That was the final salutation in an email from an administrator at Church of the Madalene in Tulsa.

As I write this, I reflect on the many small blessings that we have in life. Without them, we can become mired in a swamp of negativity that can overwhelm us. I found many blessings in the life of my oldest brother. But I also received a few while writing this book about his tragic life and death. This was one of them.

While researching Paul's life as a priest, I found that the Church of the Madalene in Tulsa had on its church website a history of the priests and deacons who had served the parish. Among the list of priests:

Rev. Paul W. Hight 1971–73

I was not only surprised to see my brother's name but also surprised by how much its being there meant. Many of the other names had become familiar: Sullivan, Dorney, Finn, Biller; however, most of the twenty-four priests listed I had never seen or met. Twenty of the entries included a photograph, including one of a longtime priest seemingly in reflective prayer. Only four had "No Image Available" above their names. Paul's was one of them. I recorded it and went on. I did not think about it again until years later when I mentioned it to my editor while talking about my frustrations over how the Tulsa diocese had seemingly wiped Paul out of its history except for a file deep in its secret archives and this one small website mention. My efforts to have Paul's name added to the necrology of priests of the Diocese of Tulsa on the Halpine Shrine at Holy Family Cathedral had failed. Ironically, his name remains on a plaque in the cathedral foyer that lists the ninety-six names of priests, nuns, and deacons who have served at Holy Family.

"Why don't you ask them to include a photo?" my editor suggested.

I reluctantly agreed. Using the form on the Madalene website, I sent an email identifying myself as Paul's brother and requesting that his photo be added to the history. That same day, I received a response:

> Yes! We would love to have a photo of Fr. Hight! There was a time Pictures were not as accessible, as they are now. I am unsure why there isn't a photo so yes it would be a great addition to our Priest wall in the library, too! Thank you again for contacting us.

The blessings salutation followed.

I found my only color photo of Paul as a priest: the Paul I remembered, in his priest's collar, smiling broadly, with those welcoming eyes. I sent it in an email the next day. Within a week, my brother's photograph had been posted—another blessing from a woman I had never met. And then, after learning of its existence from my wife, I left an intention in Holy Family Cathedral's Prayers and Petitions/In Thanksgiving book:

> The Rev. Paul W. Hight, deceased 2000.
> Served here 1973–1974.

In Loving Memory
Paul Hight

December 27, 1942 - December 14, 2000

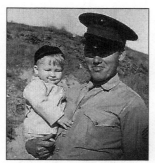

Wilber Hight with Paul, 1944

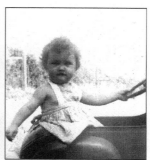

Baby Linda, summer 1948

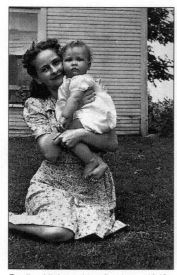

Pauline Hight and her first born, 1943

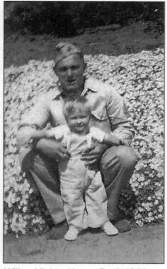

Wilber Hight with son Paul, 1944

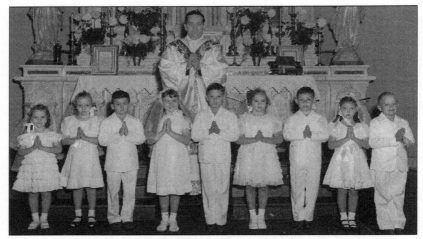

First Communion: Bishop Sullivan with Saint Mary's second-graders in Guthrie; Paul, far right

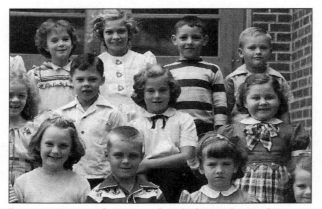

Paul, top right corner, Saint Mary's Catholic School, Guthrie, Oklahoma

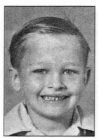 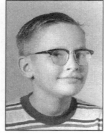 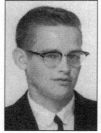 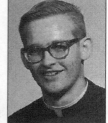

Left, Paul in grade school; right, age 10, 1952   *Paul's late teen and seminary years*

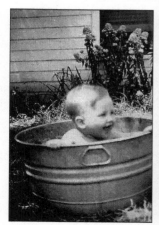

Paul bathing, summer 1943

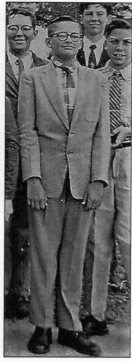

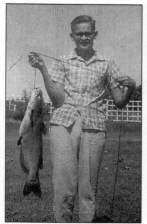

Paul and his big catfish

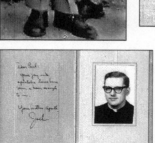

Above left, a young Paul; above right, official 1960 graduate list from Saint John's Seminary.

Left, a card from Paul's fellow Oklahoma priest Jack Petuskey

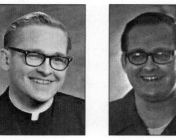

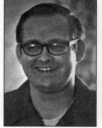

The Rev. Paul Hight through the years   *Left, Paul mid-thirties; right, post 1996 shooting*

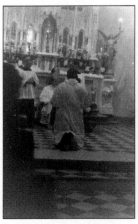
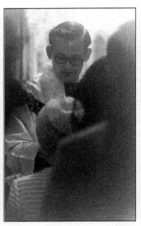
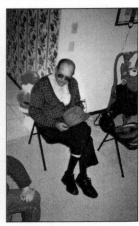

Paul's ordination, 1968   Paul giving communion, 1968   Paul's final Christmas, 1999

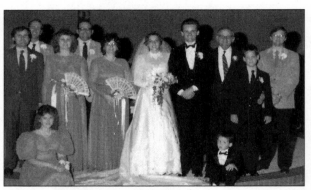

Hight clan, Joe and Nan's wedding, 1986; Paul, back row, second left

". . . unless you turn and become like children,
you will not enter the kingdom of heaven.
Whoever humbles himself like this child is
the greatest in the kingdom of heaven.
And whoever receives one child such as
this in my name receives me."
(MT 18: 2-6)

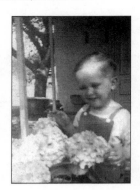

Paul Hight, age 2, at home

Acknowledgments

This book took more than a decade to complete, but it would not been possible without the help of many people.

First, my wife, Nan, and daughters, Elena and Elyse. All three encouraged me along the way to finish the book and complete the journey of understanding what had happened to Paul. They were understanding to a fault, and I am eternally grateful for them. Nan was especially patient with me when I said I could not run an errand or do something extra because I was working on the book. She also became the person who listened to me throughout the research for and completion of the book. Elena also was instrumental in reading the book, providing useful and insightful feedback, and helping me compile my notes and documents into an understandable order.

Second, my mother and father, Wilber and Pauline Hight. While they were not alive to influence this book, they were always there for me as an influence. They talked to me about the issues as best they could when they were alive. They always provided inspiration to finish what I started. They were the foundation of what a family was and should be, even in the most difficult and darkest times.

I also thank my sisters, Susan and Marilyn; brothers, John and Bill; brother-in-law, Michael Williams; and sister-in-law, Jan Hight. I tested their memory and their patience with my questions. They spurred me on by sharing details that I did not know. They also gave me insight on what I might not have understood. Other relatives, such as Kenneth McWethy and Arlene Meier, were also incredibly patient with questions asked by their cousin. They filled in many blanks about my family's early days that I would not been able to find out otherwise.

Then there's Jeanne Devlin, editor and publisher of the RoadRunner Press. Jeanne told me that she wanted a book that made a difference. She wanted a book that provided hope even through the most difficult of circumstances. I hope this book does both. Jeanne also pushed me to find additional sources that added to the book and its depth. She a great teacher and motivator—and an invaluable resource for authors.

Many priests, such as Father Joe Ross and Monsignor Dennis Dorney and the late Father Lowell Stieferman and Father Denis Hanrahan, as well as other former priests, provided insight and leads to other sources. Without question, most priests are wonderful and caring people who strive to help others in their work. They are blessings to the people they serve.

Father Elkin Gonzalez, vicar general for the Tulsa Diocese, and Joey Spencer, diocesan archivist, both came through with information or ideas that I had struggled to obtain from the diocese in the past. Both also were patient with my inquiries and helpful with their replies.

Authors Mark Masse, George Getschow, and Nancy Berland were instrumental in providing helpful tips and insight in the early stages of writing this book. Author Maria Ruiz Scaperlanda provided insight and ideas on how to proceed with certain sources within the Church. Tom Maupin, whom I consider one of the nation's best copy editors, and his wife, Marge, provided valuable input and edits toward the completion of the manuscript. The tips I also received at the Mayborn Literary Nonfiction Conference were helpful in the initial stages of the book.

I don't know how many times I called or emailed Jeffrey Dismukes, communications director of the Oklahoma Department of Mental

Health and Substance Abuse Services. He scheduled site visits and provided information, clarity, and insight in a timely manner. He told his own story. He became a trusted source whom I turned to consistently. He and Steven Buck and Michael Brose earned my respect for the people they are. I can't begin to express my appreciation to them for their help with this book.

During his tenure as chief of police for Oklahoma City (he retired in 2019), Bill Citty was one of the most respected law enforcement officials by the media, even though he might not have always agreed with what we wrote all the time. He was forthright in responding to me and considerate with most of my requests.

The Oklahoma History Center provided a wealth of information and background material. I spent three or four days there and plan to spend more on future projects. Its documents and publications are vital links to history and must continue to be protected. The archives of *The Oklahoman*, *Tulsa World*, *Oklahoma Courier*, *Guthrie Daily Leader*, and other media were also vital in my research.

Many others also were instrumental in the writing of this book. Some of them provided me with links to studies or a tidbit of information that led me to a new source. Alan Krieger, librarian for Theology, Philosophy, and Jewish Studies at the University of Notre Dame, and Jean McManus, the university's Catholic studies librarian, pointed me to important documents concerning the Catholic Church and mental illness. That caused me to research further. Sources such as these, including those unnamed people who work for a church or organization, were vital in my research and understanding.

And finally, I want to thank all of those who are continuing in their research of mental illness and the fight to end the stigma associated with it. You are the reason I have hope for a future in which people with mental illness will not have to fear authority figures or face stigma that forces them to become misfits in our society.

My brother Paul was the most important part of this book. He faced judgment and stigma many times in his life. He faced tragedy. He faced death. But in his darkest hours, he yearned for life beyond his illness. His writings were invaluable in proving that. He wrote about fear only once. He mentioned death four times. But he wrote about life and everlasting life more than twenty-five times. The one time he wrote about fear was when he was emphasizing how fear, doubt, and despair are the devil's three principal devices. He then wrote three words as complete sentences to counter evil and obtain a fuller life:

Love. Faith. Hope.

The people mentioned in these acknowledgments gave me what I needed to write this book, the love and support to continue with it, and the faith that I could finish it. I know Paul would be thankful to each of you, as I am.

Bibliography

"About Saint John the Evangelist Roman Catholic Church," http://www.St-john-mcalester.org.

"Adult Crisis Centers." Oklahoma Department of Mental Health and Substance Abuse Services, http://www.ok.gov.odmhsas.

Abram, Susan. "Jail Psych Ward Treats Sickest of Mentally Ill Inmates." *Los Angeles Daily News*, October 19, 2008, http://www.dailynews.com/20081019/jail-psych-ward-treats-sickest-of-mentally-ill-inmates.

"A Healing Agent: The Chicago Catholic Archdiocesan Commission on Mental Illness," http://www.miministry.org.

"A History of Together for Life," http://www.togetherforlifeonline.com.

"Anderson Ready To Accept Consequences of State Investigation." *Guthrie Daily Leader*, April 14, 1996.

Anthony, Chuck. "Ed Kelly, City Priest, Weds." *The Daily Oklahoman*, September 28, 1968.

Appointment of executor for Paul Wilber Hight, December 19, 2000, Oklahoma County, state of Oklahoma. Certified copy in possession of author.

Archdiocese of Oklahoma City. "An Era of Hope 1977–1991: Archbishop Charles A. Salatka: Archbishop Salatka's Years in Oklahoma," http://www.archokc.org/history/1977–1993.

———. "One Becomes Two: 1972–1977: Archbishop John R. Quinn," http://www.archokc.org/history/1972–1975.

"Assignments for 31 Priests Announced." *The Daily Oklahoman*, May 28, 1971.

"A ZENIT Daily Dispatch: Impediments to Ordination." ZENIT International

News Agency, provided courtesy of Eternal Word Television Network, http://www.ewtn.com.

Barry, Ellen. "Priest Treatment Unfolds in Costly, Secretive World." *The Boston Globe*, April 3, 2002, http://www.bostonglobe.com/news/special-rports/2002/04/02/priest-treatment-unfolds-costly-secretive-world/deAcdZXnaXuLvHcPbNip7L/story.html.

Beal, John P., ed. "Minor Seminaries." *New Commentary on the Code of Canon Law*, study edition. Mahwah, New Jersey: Paulist Press, January 1, 2000.

Begley, Sharon. "The Schizophrenic Mind." *Newsweek*, March 11, 2002.

"Benztropine MESYLATE," http://www.webmd.com.

Bickham, Jack M. "Board Uncertain: Priests Gloomy." *The Oklahoma Courier*, September 20, 1968.

"Bishop's Installation Is Awaited." *Grand Island Independent*, September 20, 1972.

"Bishop To Ordain Guthrian." *Guthrie Daily Leader*, n.d.

"Bishops Urged To Sponsor Study." *The Oklahoma Courier*, April 15, 1968.

"Bishop Reed Known as a 'Liberal.' " *The Oklahoma Journal*, January 4, 1972.

"Bishop Reed To Attend U. S. Group Session." *The Oklahoma Courier*, April 12, 1968.

Bland, Karina. "Budget Faulted in Boy's Death: With No Treatment Funds, Juveniles Go To Jail." *The Arizona Republic*, July 17, 2002.

Bogan, Jesse. "Along with Business, History and Legends Crowd Saint Louis Police HQ." *Saint Louis Post-Dispatch*, January 30, 2011.

Bonner, Jeremy. *The Road to Renewal: Victor Joseph Reed & Oklahoma Catholicism*, 1905–1971. Washington, D.C.: Catholic University of America Press, 2008.

Booth, William. "Texas Primer: The Stock Tank." *Texas Monthly*, May 1986.

"Canon Law." United States Conference of Catholic Bishops, http://usccb.org.

Capps, Sarah. "Continuity in Care: The History of Deinstitutionalization in Oklahoma's Mental Healthcare System." University of Oklahoma, honors thesis, 2015, http: http://www.ou.edu/content/dam/cas/history/docs/journal/02_Capps_-_Continuity_in_Care_for_publication.pdf.

Cassock, The. Saint Louis, Missouri: Cardinal Glennon College, May 1963.

Catholic Bishops of the United States. "Responsibility, Rehabilitation, and Restoration: A Catholic Perspective on Crime and Criminal Justice." Washington, D.C.: United States Conference of Catholic Bishops, 2000, http://www.usccb.org/issues-and-action/human-life-and-dignity/criminal-justice-restorative-justice/crime-and-criminal-justice.cfm.

"Catholic Church Assignments Made." *McAlester News-Capital*, June 3, 1968.

"Catholic Entry in State Council Eyed." *The Oklahoma Courier*, March 29, 1968.

Catholic Hierarchy. "Archbishop Eusebius Joseph Beltran," http://www.catholic-hierarchy.org/bishop/bbeltran.html.

——. "Archbishop John Raphael Quinn," http://www.catholic-hierarchy.org/bishop/bquinn.html.

——. "Bishop Bernard James Ganter," http://www.catholic-hierarchy.org/bishop/bganter.html.

——. "Bishop John Joseph Sullivan," http://www.catholic-hierarchy.org/bishop/bsullj.html.

——. "Diocese of Tulsa," http://www.catholic-hierarchy.org/diocese/dtuls.html.

——. "The Year of Our Lord 1968," http://www.catholic-hierarchy.org/events/y1968.html.

"Chaplain Named at Hillcrest." *Tulsa Daily World*, May 28, 1971.

"Celebrating the 10th anniversary of Bishop John J. Sullivan in the Diocese of Kansas City–Saint Joseph," *The Catholic Key,* vol. 19, no. 23, August 16, 1987.

——. Sly, Julie. "So what's a bishop's life like anyway?"

——. "Growth in ministry marks bishop's tenure."

——. "A bishop has to be very personal."

Storms, Mary Pat. "Those who know him describe Bishop Sullivan."

Church of the Madalene. "Madalene History," http://www.madalenetulsa.org/Madalene-History.

"Closure of Courier on April 11." *The Oklahoma Courier*, February 21, 1969.

Clay, Nolan, and Bryan Dean. "Former Oklahoma County DA Macy Dies." *The Oklahoman*, November 19, 2011.

Cochran, Sam. "CIT Training: October 29–November 2, 2001." Memphis, Tennessee: Memphis Police Department Crisis Intervention Team, August 29, 2001.

Cohen, Jennie. "7 Surprising Facts about Joan of Arc," January 28, 2013, http://www.history.com.

Corovessis, Babs. "Controversial State Priest Takes Bride." *The Daily Oklahoman*, June 4, 1968.

Craughwell, Thomas J. *Patron Saints: Saints for Every Member of Your Family, Every Profession, Every Ailment, Every Emergency, and Even Every Amusement*. Huntington, Indiana: Our Sunday Visitor Publishing Division, 2011.

Dahl, Julia. "How To Stop Suicide by Cop." *Miller-McCune Magazine*. The Investigative Fund, the Nation Institute, February 24, 2011.

Dan Allen Center for Social Justice. "Projects," http://www.danallencenter.org/index.php?id=projects.

"Deadly Force: Threat Response Plan Should Be Reviewed." *The Daily Oklahoman*, December 24, 2000.

"Death Row Full; No Executions Expected." Associated Press. *McAlester News-Capital*, June 12, 1969.

"Delegates' Zeal Promises Bright Future for Little Council." *The Oklahoma Courier*, April 26, 1968.

"Diocese's 5th Bishop is Young Man of 42." *The Oklahoma Journal*, January 4, 1972.

Diocese of Tulsa. "A Brief History of the Diocese," https://www.dioceseoftulsa.

org/a-brief-history-of-the-diocese.

Diocese of Tulsa Directory, 1974.

Diocese of Tulsa Directory, 1976.

Eaglet, The: "Class of '60." San Antonio, Texas: Saint John's Seminary, 1960.

"Eastern State Hospital," http://www.AbandonOK.com.

"Ecclesial Movements: The Catholic Charismatic Renewal," http://www.catholic. org.

"Eighth Sunday of Ordinary Time." Sunday Bulletin 30, no. 30. Hennessey, Oklahoma: Church of Saint Joseph, 2000.

"Ex-Logan County Sheriff, 81, Dies," March 2, 2010, http://www.NewsOK.com.

"Experimental Mass Approved." *The Oklahoma Courier*, n.d.

"Father Caldwell Quits Priesthood." *The Oklahoma Courier*, n.d.

"Father Kenneth King, a Priest 50 Years, Dies at 76." Roman Catholic Diocese of Tulsa, last modified July 11, 2007, http://www.dioceseoftulsa.org/article. asp?nID=97.

"54 Assignments of Diocesan Priests Listed." *The Oklahoma Courier*, June 7, 1968.

First Capitol Apartments, 1600 East College Avenue, Guthrie, Logan County, Oklahoma, http://www.affordablehousingonline.com.

"First Contact—The Street Officer: Dealing with People Who Exhibit Abnormal Behavior." Madison, Wisconsin: NAMI Wisconsin., n.d.

Florida Partners in Crisis, http://www.floridapartnersincrisis.org.

Ford, Brian. "House Approves Funds for Mental Health Terms." *Tulsa World*, May 11, 2001.

"Former District Attorney To Be Released from Prison." *Daily O'Collegian*, Oklahoma State University, September 4, 1997.

"Former Nun Weds Merchant." Associated Press. *McAlester News-Capital*, June 12, 1969.

"For the Lonely and Despairing, a Haven of Hope Becomes a Reality in Tulsa." *The Oklahoma Courier,* April 12, 1968.

"42 CFR Part 2—Confidentiality of Alcohol and Drug Abuse Patient Records," http://www.law.cornell.edu.

FY-2004 budget request prioritization. Oklahoma Department of Mental Health and Substance Abuse Services, September 16, 2002.

Gable, Kelly, and Daniel Carlat. "Long Acting Injectable Antipsychotics: A Primer," http://www.pro.psychcentral.com.

Gaalaas, Monsignor Patrick, interview by author Joe Hight, April 10, 2019.

"Genetic Clues Hold Key to Schizophrenia Treatment." *Science Daily*, March 24, 2009, https://www.sciencedaily.com/releases/2009/03/090319224552.htm.

Godfrey, Ed. "Fatal Shooting of Man Justified, Macy Rules." *The Daily Oklahoman*, December 30, 2000.

Gold, Jenny. "San Antonio Police Have Radical Approach to Mental Illness:

Treat It." Kaiser Health News, August 19, 2014, http://www.NewsOK.com.

"Gunshot Wound to the Abdomen," http://www.drug.com.

Gust, Steve. "Archdiocesan Priests Celebrate 50 Years of Service to God." *Sooner Catholic*, August 30, 2009.

"Guthrie Man Shot During Altercation." *Guthrie Daily Leader*, April 9, 1996.

"Haldol Injection for Intramuscular Injection Only, Production Information," http://www.janssen.com.

Hall, Richard. "12 of Oklahoma's beautifully creepy abandoned places, part 2," October 31, 2013, http://www.NewsOK.com.

"Haloperidol (Haldol)," National Alliance on Mental Illness, http://www.name.org.

Harper, David. "Slain Teen's Family Wins Suit." *Tulsa World*, March 31, 2000.

Havlik, Bernard J., J.C.L., Open letter to the Oklahoma City–Tulsa diocese, *The Oklahoma Courier*, n.d.

Havorka, Jack, letter to author Joe Hight, May 9, 1986.

Helman, Scott. "The San Antonio Way: How One Texas City Took on Mental Health as a Community—and Became a National Model." *The Boston Globe*, December 10, 2016.

Herndon, Jennie, letter to author Joe Hight, Oklahoma City, Oklahoma, n.d.

Hegyi, Vladimir. Hegyi. "Dermatologic Manifestations of Pellagra Differential Diagnoses," https://emedicine.medscape.com/article/1095845-differential.

Hight, Joe. "Winning Isn't Everything . . . But It Sure Is Nice!" *Et Al.*, vol. 1, no. 2, fall-winter 1978.

——. "Brain-Damaged Baby Has 'Purpose.' " *The Shawnee News-Star*, October 6, 1984.

——. "Letter to Catholic Young Adults." Young Adult Ministry—Oklahoma Style, 5, December 1985, 2–3.

——. "Mother Leaves Legacy of Love to Her Family." *The Daily Oklahoman*, May 9, 1986.

——. Obituary for Paul Hight. *The Daily Oklahoman*, December 17, 2000.

——. "Story in Oklahoman." Email to Michael Brose, May 17, 2001.

——. "The Voices That Stalked a Roman Catholic Priest." Speech, Georgetown University, Washington, D.C., 2008.

Hight, Paul. "Backfire!" *The Cassock*, n.d.. 14–17.

Hinton, Mick. "House Approves Programs To Help Mentally Ill People." *The Oklahoman*, May 11, 2001.

——. "Aid Sought for Mentally Ill." *The Oklahoman*, July 15, 2002.

"History of the Casa." The Pontifical North American College, http://www.pnac.org.

"Holloway, William Judson (1888–1970)." Oklahoma Historical Society, http://www.okhistory.org.

"How Schizophrenia Develops: New Evidence and New Ideas." *The Harvard Health Letter*, vol. 17, no. 8, February 2001, 1–4.

"Impediments to Ordination." Irondale, Alabama: Eternal Word Television Network, February 7, 2012, http://www.ewtn.com.

"Introduction to the Sermon on Mount," Bible Gateway, http://biblegateway.com.

"Irked Cardinal Warns Priests in Washington." *The Oklahoma Courier*, September 6, 1968.

James, J. Frank, and Dick Gregory. "Improving Psychiatric Care for Prisoners." *Hospital & Community Psychiatry*, vol. 31, no. 10, October 1980, 671–673.

James, J. Frank, Dick Gregory, Renee K. Jones, and O. H. Rundell. "Psychiatric Morbidity in Prisons." *Hospital & Community Psychiatry*, vol. 31, no. 10, October 1980, 674–677.

Jarrett, Lew. "A Job To Be Done: Views of Tulsa's North Side." *The Oklahoma Courier*, June 21, 1968.

Jibson, Michael D., and Rajiv Tandon. "New Atypical Antipsychotic Medications." *Journal of Psychiatric Research*, 32, 1998, 215–228.

"Joe Mendosa." Oklahoma Department of Corrections.

John Paul II, Pope. "Mentally Ill Are Also Made in God's Image." *L'Osservatore Romano*, December 11, 1996, https://www.ewtn.com/library/PAPALDOC/JP96N30.htm.

Keeping, Juliana. "Deadly Force: A Decade of Oklahoma City Police Department Shootings," May 11, 2014, The Oklahoman/NewsOK.com.

Kenrick-Glennon Seminary. "History of the Seminary," http://kenrick.edu/about/history-of-kenrick-glennon-seminary/.

Khandaker, Golam M., Jorge Zimbron, and Peter B. Jones. "Childhood Infection and Adult Schizophrenia: A Meta-analysis of Population-based Studies." *Schizophrenia Research*, June 15, 2012. https://www.ncbi.nlm.nih.gov/pubmed/22704639.

Kliewar, Stephen P., Melissa McNally, and Robyn L. Trippany. "Deinstitutionalization: Its Impact on Community Mental Health Centers and the Seriously Mentally Ill." Walden University, *The Alabama Counseling Association Journal*, vol. 35, no. 1., 2009. https://files.eric.ed.gov/fulltext/EJ875402.pdf.

Lackmeyer, Steve. "Man's Mental State Questioned." *The Daily Oklahoman*, April 18, 1996.

——. "City's New Police Chief Facing Tight Budget, Aging Fleet." *The Daily Oklahoman*, March 3, 1998.

"Laicization Explained by Archbishop." *The Oklahoma Courier*, February 21, 1969.

"Laicization (Loss of Clerical State)." *New Catholic Encyclopedia*, Catholic University of America. Washington, D.C.: Thomson/Gale Group, 2003.

Langford, Mary Diane. "Shepherd in the Image of Christ: The Centennial History of Saint John's–Assumption Seminary, San Antonio, Texas," 2014.

Lattin, Don. "Archbishop Quinn of S. F. to Resign: His Successor Is a Conservative." *San Francisco Gate*, August 16, 1995, http://www.sfgate.com/news/article/PAGE-ONE-Archbishop-Quinn-of-S-F-To-Resign-3026218.php.

"Logan County Hospital," http://www.AbandonOK.com.

Lowery, Wesley, Kimberly Kindy, Keith L. Alexander, Julie Tate, Jennifer Jenkins, and Steven Rich. "Distraught People, Deadly Results: Officers Often Lack the Training To Approach the Mentally Unstable, Experts Say." *The Washington Post*, June 30, 2015.

Lucas, Lisa. "Changing the Way Police Respond to Mental Illness," September 28, 2016, http://www.CNN.com.

"Major Issues Face General Assembly Session Next Week." *The Oklahoma Courier*, April 12, 1968.

Malcom, Mike. "Shrine for Deceased Priests Blessed: Bishop Slattery Blessed Halpine Shine in November." Holy Family Cathedral. *Cathedral News*, vol. 19, no. 5, 2014.

"Man Charged in Mom's Death." *The Oklahoman*, April 26, 1995, http://www.newsok.com/article/2500163.

"Man with Knife Killed by Police." ChannelOklahoma.com, December 15, 2000.

Martin, Linda. "Man Admits Guilt in Mother's Murder." *Tulsa World*, February 28, 1996.

May, Doyle. "Key Issues To Be Aired at Assembly." *The Oklahoma Courier*, April 19, 1968.

———. "Little Council OK's Reforms, Rejects Money-spending Ideas." *The Oklahoma Courier*, April 26, 1968.

———. "A Report on Tulsa's North Side." *The Oklahoma Courier*, June 21, 1968.

McCarthy, John. "Bishop Emeritus John McCarthy: A Reflection on 60 Years of Change." *Austin American-Statesmen*, May 25, 2016, http://www.mystatesman.com/news/opinion/bishop-emeritus-john-mccarthy-reflection-years-change/xQXWliFxlali2JZv1IHnGM/.

———. "No Shame in Mental Illness." A Bishop's Blog—Common Sense Catholicism, February 15, 2013, http://www.bishopjohnmccarthy.com/tag/mental-illness/.

McNutt, Michael. "Ex-Prosecutor Gets Two-year Prison Sentence: Anderson Says He Blames Himself." *The Daily Oklahoman*, October 29, 1996.

"Medical Record Retention Required of Health Care Providers: 50 State Comparison." Health Information & the Law Project, Milken Institute School of Public Health, George Washington University, http://www.healthinfolaw.org.

Medley, Robert. "After Shooting, Police Prepare for Stun Guns." *The Daily Oklahoman*, August 23, 2001.

———. "Norman 'Connections' Closing: Residents May Be Moved to City." *The Daily Oklahoman*, September 6, 1996.

"Memphis Police Crisis Intervention Team." Booklet, city of Memphis, Tennessee, 1999.

"Mental Health Services for Oklahoma Prisons." Oklahoma City, Oklahoma: Oklahoma Department of Mental Health, 1979.

"Exhibition Overview: Heavenly Bodies: Fashion and the Catholic Imagination." New York: Metropolitan Museum of Art, May 10–October 8, 2018, http://www.metmuseum.org, visited by author Joe Hight, June 3, 2018.

Meyer, Ali. "Exclusive: Inside the Oklahoma Hospital for the Insane." KFOR-TV, May 20, 2015, http://www.kfor.com.

Money, Jack. "Services Set for Priest Who Aided Refugees." March 31, 1990, http://www.NewsOK.com.

Money, Jack, and Steve Lackmeyer. "Citizen Review Board Not a Magic Bullet." *The Daily Oklahoman*, October 25, 1999.

Moore, Sylvia. "Seaside To Pay Vaughns." *The Herald*, January 5, 2001.

——. "Vaughn Family Heading toward Recovery." *The Herald*, January 6, 2001.

"Morbidity and Mortality Weekly Report." Centers for Disease Control and Prevention, http://www.cdc.gov.

"Most Priests Who Resigned Cite Celibacy." *The Oklahoma Courier*, n.d.

Morelli, Brad, interviewed by author Joe Hight, December 10, 2018.

Morgan, Father Martin, interview by author Joe Hight, April 13, 2019.

Murray, Alan. "If Bioterror Hit U. S., Would Public Know How to Stay Safe?" *Wall Street Journal*, October 15, 2002.

"National Catholic Partnership on Disability/Mental Illness," http://www.ncpd.org.

"Nebraska Bishops' Statements on Affirming the Dignity of the Mentally Ill." Nebraska Catholic Conference, last modified February 2005, http://www.necatholic.org/Websites/nebcathcon/files/Content/5439572/Bishops_Statement--Affirming_the_Dignity_of_the_Mentally_Ill.pdf.

Neill, Steve. "Bishop Invites Priests Who Left Voluntarily To Return to Ministry or Seek Laicization." *The Catholic Virginian*, March 4, 2008, http://www.catholic.org/lent/story.php?id=27065..

Nelson, Mary Jo. "The 1980s 10 Turbulent Years." *The Daily Oklahoman*, December 31, 1989.

NC News Service, "Resignations of 463 priests in 1968 listed." *The Oklahoma Courier*, September 1968.

New American Bible, Saint Joseph edition. New York: Catholic Book Publishing Co., 1970.

"New Assistant Pastor on Staff at Saint John's." *McAlester News-Capital*, June 18, 1968.

New York State Catholic Conference. " 'For I Am Lonely and Afflicted': Toward a Just Response to the Needs of Mentally Ill Persons," last modified February 4, 2014, http://www.nyscatholic.org/2014/02/for-i-am-lonely-and-afflicted/.

Nomani, Asra Q. "My Brother's Battle—and Mine." *The Washington Post*, April 29, 2007, http://www.washingtonpost.com/wp-dyn/content/article/2007/04/27/AR2007042702053.html.

"Norman State Hospital," http://www.asylumprojects.org.

"Nuncio." *New Advent*, http://www.newadvent.org.

"Nuptials Held for Three Pairs." *The Daily Oklahoman*, July 15, 1972.

"Oil Embargo 1973–1974." Office of Historian: Milestones: 1969–1976, History.

"OCU Honors Bishop Reed." *The Oklahoma Courier*, May 10, 1968.

"OKC Sees Rash of Police Involved Shootings." ChannelOklahoma.com, December 6, 2000.

Ordinary People, Extraordinary Lives: Inspirational Stories of the Saints, IMP Inc., n.d.

Our Sunday's Visitors Encyclopedia of Saints Revised. Huntington, Indiana: Our Sunday Visitor Publishing Division, 2003.

Parker, Laurence. Letter to the editor. *Guthrie Daily Leader*, April 9, 1996.

Parks, Joe, and Peggy Jewell, eds. *Technical Report on Smoking Policy and Treatment in State Operated Psychiatric Facilities*. National Association of State Mental Health Program Directors, Medical Directors Council, October 2006.

"Pastoral Board Asks Clergy for Pay Plan." *The Oklahoma Courier*, n.d.

Patton, Ann. "What People Are Saying about Dan's War on Poverty: A Grassroots Crusade for Social Justice," http://annpatton.net/dans-war-on-poverty/reviews/.

Perlin, Michael L. "Half-wracked Prejudice Leaped Forth: Sanism, Pretextuality, and Why and How Mental Disability Law Developed as It Did." *Journal of Contemporary Legal Issues*, 10, 1999, 3–36.

Peters, Edward N., curator. *The 1917 Pio-Benedictine Code of Canon Law*, in English translation with extensive scholarly apparatus. San Francisco: Ignatius Press, September 1, 2001.

Phillips, Mark. "Tulsa Throng Mourns Reed." *The Daily Oklahoman*, September 12, 1971.

Plumberg, Diane, and Steve Lackmeyer. "Police Chief Job Going to Deputy: 27-year Officer To Lead Force." *The Daily Oklahoman*, February 28, 1998.

Poggioli, Sylvia. "Vatican II: A Half-century Later, a Mixed Legacy." NPR Europe, October 11, 2012.

"Police Chief Reacts to Recent Killings." ChannelOklahoma.com, December 21, 2000.

"Police Consider 'Non-Lethal' Alternatives." ChannelOklahoma.com, December 15, 2000.

"Police Shooting Victim Had Mental Illness." ChannelOklahoma.com, December 15, 2000.

"Pope Francis Appoints Father David Konderla as Fourth Bishop of Tulsa, OK." Saint Mary Cathedral, Catholic Diocese of Austin, May 13, 2016.

"Positive Signs Seen in Crisis of Church," NC News Service, *The Oklahoma Courier*, March 28, 1969.

Poston, Ben. "Choice as Bishop Shock to Tulsan." *The Daily Oklahoman*, July 26, 1972.

"Questions and Answers: On Being Dismissed from Clerical State." *The Catholic Sun*, February 16, 2010, http://www.catholicsun.org.

Rabalais, Celie. "City Police Shoot, Kill Knife-wielding Suspect." *The Daily Oklahoman*, December 15, 2000.

Rashke, Richard. *The Killing of Karen Silkwood: The Story Behind the Kerr-McGee Plutonium Case*. Ithaca, New York: ILR Press, 1981.

Raymond, Ken. "Police Kill Mental Patient." *The Daily Oklahoman*, December 16, 2000.

———. "City Council Restricts Police Pursuit, Amends Policies." *The Daily Oklahoman*, August 15, 2001.

———. "Crisis Team Helps Police Deal with Mentally Ill." The Oklahoman/NewsOK.com, April 8, 2002, http://www.newsok.com.

———. "Stories of the Ages: Endangered Black History: Guthrie Has Lost Pieces of its Black History, but Remains a Vital Community." *The Oklahoman*, January 28, 2012.

Redemptorist Fathers of Okmulgee. "An Interview with Bishop Reed." Insert to *The Oklahoma Courier*, March 1968.

Reid, Jim. "Racial Causes Behind Zoning Rule, He Says: Church, Others Claim Officials Show Prejudice." *The Daily Oklahoman*, January 29, 1969.

Reinstatement of Paul R. Anderson to membership in the Oklahoma Bar Association and to the roll of attorneys. Oklahoma Supreme Court, July 2, 2002.

Report of investigation of medical examiner on Paul Hight, Board of Medicolegal Investigations, Office of the Chief Medical Examiner, filed by Dr. Jeffery Gofton, December 15, 2000.

Rettner, Rachael. "Colorado Survivors: How Do People Survive Gunshot Wounds?" *LiveScience*, July 23, 2012.

Reverend Denis Hanrahan obituary, Smith & Kernke Funeral Homes & Crematory, March 20, 2016, http://www.smithandkernke.com.

"San Antonio Missions," National Park Service, http://www.nps.gov.

Saxon, Wolfgang. "Rev. Joseph H. Fichter, 85, Dies: A Jesuit Sociologist and Professor," *The New York Times*, February 26, 1994.

Scaperlanda, Maria Ruiz. *The Shepherd Who Didn't Run: Father Stanley Rother, Martyr from Oklahoma*. Huntington, Indiana: Our Sunday Visitor Inc., 2015.

"Schizophrenia Facts and Statistics," http://www.schizophrenia.com.

Schlect, Dean. "Brief Biography," http://www.deanschlecht.com/about.html, 2017.

Schneider, Keith. "Rash of Suicides in Oklahoma Shows That the Crisis on the Farm Goes On." *The New York Times*, August 17, 1987.

Seper, Cardinal Franjo. "The Role of Women in Modern Society and the Church." Sacred Congregation for the Doctrine of the Faith, October 15, 1976, Vatican.va.

"72 Priests in Diocese Oppose Encyclical." *The Oklahoma Courier*, August 16, 1968.

Sherman, Bill. "Catholic Church Building Shrine to Mexican Saint." *Tulsa*

World, August 16, 2014, TulsaWorld.com.

Shoemaker, Sharlene. "Neighbor for Neighbor." *The Oklahoma Courier*, February 14, 1969.

Sly, Julie. "So What's a Bishop's Life Like Anyway?: To Carry Out His Ministry, He Must Be with the People." *The Catholic Key*, August 16, 1987.

"Son Handed Life Term in Slaying." *The Daily Oklahoman*, May 1, 1996.

Spearman, C. H. Jr., *God Isn't Through with Me*. Edmond, Oklahoma: Spearman Publishing Company, Inc., 1999.

"State Catholic Church Division Line Set." *The Daily Oklahoman*, December 23, 1972.

"Stillwater Priest Quits to Marry." *The Daily Oklahoman*, May 8, 1973.

Sullivan, John Joseph. Interview. *The Catholic Key*, August 16, 1987.

——. "This Was Not Simply My Vision, but Our Vision." *The Catholic Key*, August 16, 1987.

"Supermarket Only Holdout in Boycott by Tulsa Blacks." *The Daily Oklahoman*, August 8, 1971.

Sutter, Ellie. "Longtime Guthrie Doctor Dies." *The Daily Oklahoman*, June 19, 1992.

Tatum, Lisa. "Oklahoma Native Appointed Mental Health Commissioner." *The Daily Oklahoman*, January 13, 2001.

Teicher, Jordan G. "Why Is Vatican II So Important?" National Public Radio, October 10, 2012, http://www.npr.org/2012/10/10/162573716/why-is-vatican-ii-so-important.

Terry, Karen J. "The Causes and Context of Sexual Abuse of Minors by Catholic Priests in the United States, 1950–2010." John Jay College Research Team, May 2011. Available from United States Conference of Catholic Bishops, http://www.usccb.org/issues-and-action/child-and-youth-protection/upload/The-Causes-and-Context-of-Sexual-Abuse-of-Minors-by-Catholic-Priests-in-the-United-States-1950-2010.pdf.

"Timeline: Deinstitutionalization and Its Consequences," *Mother Jones*, April 29, 2013.

The Jerusalem Bible. New York: Doubleday & Company, 1966.

"The Problem: Functionary Priest." Religious News Service. *The Oklahoma Courier*, May 17, 1968.

"The Vatican II—Voice of the Church," http://www.vatican2voice.org.

Thornton, Anthony. "Former DA Behind Bars, But Not for Long." *The Daily Oklahoman*, January 1997.

"Top 10 Forms of Psychiatric Institution Abuse." The Mental Health Watchdog. CCHR International, November 12, 2014, http://www.cchrint.org.

TOPICC: The Oklahoma Partnership in Creating Change. "Mission," http://www.metaicon.com/clients/topicc/mission.htm.

Torrey, E. Fuller. "Ronald Reagan's Shameful Legacy: Violence, the Homeless, Mental Illness." *Salon Magazine*, September 29, 2013.

"Prison Issues Grow in Size and Complexity." Treatment Advocacy Center, Date of publication? http://www.treatmentadvocacycenter.org.

"Tulsa Catholic Center Folds Its Newspaper." *The Oklahoma Courier*, April 12, 1968.

"Tulsa, City Rites Planned for Reed." *The Daily Oklahoman*, September 9, 1971.

"Tulsa Diocese Reports Seven Clergy Accused." *The Oklahoman*, February 19, 2004, http://newsok.com/article/1890586.

"Tulsan To Become Bishop." *The Daily Oklahoman*, September 19, 1972.

Turner, Paul. "Priestly People: A Look at Holy Orders, Celibacy, Training, Other Topics," http://paulturner.org/wp-content/uploads/2012/08/priesthood.htm.

"Two Named Episcopal Vicars." *The Oklahoma Courier*, February 28, 1969.

"Two Ordinations Slated." *The Oklahoma Courier*, n.d.

"2,000 See Ordination Rite." Associated Press, September 20, 1972.

Van Nuys, David. "An Interview with Thomas Joiner, Ph.D., on Why People Commit Suicide." Gulf Blend Center, http://www.gulfbend.org/poc/view_doc.php?type=doc&id=29060.

Walsh, Michael, ed. *Butler's Lives of the Saints*. New York City: HarperCollins, 1991.

"Weather History for Guthrie, OK, Guthrie Municipal," Wunderground.com. http://www.wunderground.com.

Weir, Kristin. "Smoking and Mental Illness: People with Behavioral Health Conditions Are More Likely to Smoke: Psychologists Are Among Those Working To Understand Why and Helping Them To Quit." *American Psychologist*, vol. 44, no. 6, 2013, 36.

———. "Science Watch: Smoking and Mental Illness." American Psychological Society, June 2013, http://www.apa.org.

White, James D. *The Souls of the Just: A Necrology of the Catholic Church in Oklahoma*. Tulsa, Oklahoma: The Sarton Press, 1983.

———. Tulsa: *This Far by Faith 1875–2000: 125 Years of Catholic Life in Oklahoma*: Editions du Signe, 2001.

" 'Why No Negro Homes in Edmond?' " *The Oklahoma Courier*, August 14, 1968.

"Wife of Man Shot by Police Speaks Out." ChannelOklahoma.com, November 22, 2000.

Wirth, Eileen. "People Top Priority for New G. I. Bishop." *The Oklahoma Courier*, September 22, 1972.

Zeaman, Janeice. "Archdiocese's First Bishop Installed in City." *The Daily Oklahoman*, February 7, 1973.

Zizzo, David. "Hidden Oklahoma: Norman Hospital Once a Mythical City." *The Oklahoman*, March 13, 2011.

———. "Hidden Oklahoma: 1909 Annual Report on Norman Asylum." *The Oklahoman*, March 13, 2011.

Author's Note

Numerous interviews were conducted by me in the preparation of this book. A list of the documents and materials used to create the book's narrative will be available on my author website, www.JoeHight.net.

About the Author

Joe Hight is a journalist, writer, and educator who has spent his life in the pursuit of ways and stories to help people and improve their lives. A founder of the Dart Center for Journalism and Trauma, Columbia University, New York City, Hight was editor of the *The Gazette* in Colorado Springs, Colorado, when the newspaper brought home the Pulitzer Prize in 2014. He holds the endowed chair of journalism ethics at the University of Central Oklahoma. He and his family own Best of Books in Edmond, Oklahoma.